MW00627184

THE DIETARY CURE FOR ACNE

BY
LOREN CORDAIN, PH.D.

AUTHOR OF "THE PALEO DIET" AND
"THE PALEO DIET FOR ATHLETES"

ON THE WEB AT: WWW.DIETARYACNECURE.COM

OR AT: WWW.THEPALEODIET.COM

Notice

This book is intended as a reference volume only, not as a medical manual. The information given here is designed to help you make informed decisions about your health. It is not intended as a substitute for any treatment that may have been prescribed by your doctor. If you suspect that you have a medical problem, we urge you to seek competent medical help.

Mention of specific companies, organizations, or authorities in this book does not imply endorsement by the author, nor does mention of specific companies, organizations, or authorities imply that they endorse this book.

© 2006 by Loren Cordain

All rights reserved. No part of this publication may be reproduced or transmitted in any form by any means, electronic or mechanical, including photocopying, recording, or any other information storage and retrieval system, without the written permission of the author.

Internet addresses given in this book were accurate at the time it went to press. For more information about the concepts outlined in this book visit www.thedietaryacnecure.com or at www.thepaleodiet.com

Printed in the United States of America

Published by Paleo Diet Enterprises, Fort Collins, CO

Cover design by Jason Rice

Library of Congress Cataloging-in-Publication Data
Cordain, Loren.
    The dietary cure for acne / Loren Cordain
        p.   cm
    Includes bibliographical references and index.
    ISBN-0-9785109-0-9 e-book
    ISBN-0-9785109-1-7 paperback
    1. High –protein diet. 2. Acne—Nutrition I. Title
    RM237.65.C65   2006
                    2006903539

Contents

THE AUTHOR

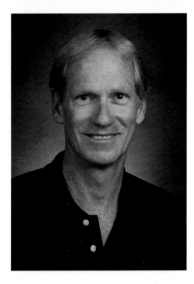

Dr. Cordain received his Ph.D. in Health from the University of Utah in 1981 and has been employed as a Professor in the Department of Health and Exercise Science at Colorado State University for the past 26 years.

Featured on Dateline NBC, the front page of the Wall Street journal, and the New York Times, Loren Cordain is widely acknowledged as one of the world's leading experts on the natural human diet of our Stone Age ancestors. He is the author of more than 100 peer-review scientific articles and abstracts. His research into the health benefits of Stone Age Diets for contemporary people has appeared in the world's top scientific journals including the American Journal of Clinical Nutrition, the British Journal of Nutrition, and the European Journal of Clinical Nutrition among others. Dr. Cordain's popular book, "The Paleo Diet" [John Wiley & Sons, 2002], has been widely acclaimed in both the scientific and lay communities and has been translated into both Danish and Swedish language versions. His follow-up book, "The Paleo Diet for Athletes" [Rodale Press], was published in November 2005.

Most recently his work has focused upon the harmful health effects of the high dietary glycemic load that is ever-present in the typical western diet and how it adversely affects skin health. In Dr. Cordain's groundbreaking paper, "Acne Vulgaris: A Disease of Western Civilization", which appeared in the prestigious medical journal, "The Archives of Dermatology", he was able to show how acne was completely absent in remote societies living and eating in a non-westernized manner.

Further, his most recent scientific paper, "Implications for the Role of Diet in Acne" outlines the underlying mechanisms of how diet causes acne.

He is the 2002 recipient of the Scholarly Excellence Award at Colorado State University for his contributions into understanding optimal human nutrition. In May of 2004 the American College for Advancement in Medicine (ACAM) recognized him with their annual "Denham Harmon Lecture" for the most significant international medical publication, "Hyperinsulinemic Diseases of Civilization: More Than Just Syndrome X". This paper represented the second in a series of his three scientific publications outlining the central role diet plays in causing acne. Dr. Cordain has spoken extensively to both the scientific and lay communities on the underlying role of diet in causing acne including invited lectures to the largest, most prestigious Dermatology Organization in the United States, The Society for Investigative Dermatology (SID) and its equivalent in Europe, The European Society of Dermatology and Venerology (EADV).

THE BOOK

The book is arranged into seven easy-to-read chapters that are fully documented by 174 scientific references. At the end of each chapter is a "BOTTOM LINE" section which summarizes the key points.

1

Overview of Acne and Diet

WHAT YOUR PHYSICIAN OR DERMATOLOGIST WILL SAY

If you were to walk into your physician's or dermatologist's office today with a full-blown case of blackheads and zits all over your face and ask them what causes this disease, you might be told, "I don't know". I quote a recent (2003) scientific review paper by Drs. Harper and Thiboutot examining the origins of acne: "despite years of research, the basic cause of acne remains unknown". If you were to press your doctor a bit further and ask them if diet causes your bad complexion, most would likely tell you that diet has virtually nothing to do with acne. In the current scientific and medical literature comments such as, "the association of diet with acne has traditionally been relegated to the category of myth", are commonplace.

Let's dig a little bit deeper. Go ahead and ask your dermatologist how they know that diet does not cause acne. They may scratch their heads a bit, rumple their brows and just give you some short answer, or even pull down one of the major textbooks on dermatology and open it up to page so and so and say, "see it says right here in this medical textbook of dermatology that diet doesn't cause acne". For most of us that would clinch it, and we would walk right out of the doctor's office thinking that diet indeed has nothing to do with acne.

THE FIRST CLUE

About 10 years ago, I hadn't really given much thought to whether or not diet could cause acne. I had pretty much assumed the party line (that diet and acne were unrelated) was correct – that is, until the day when I finally got around to reading an obscure scientific paper written by Dr. Otto Schaefer called, "When the Eskimo Comes to Town".

Dr. Schaefer was a frontier physician who treated the Inuit (Eskimo) people in remote villages and outposts from the late 1940s until the early 1970s. During this 30 year span, Dr. Schaefer observed the Inuit as they literally were transformed from the Stone Age to the space age. When he started his practice, most of the Inuit in remote areas lived and ate in the traditional manner of their ancestors dating back thousands of years. Their diet consisted almost entirely of wild animals obtained from hunting and fishing and the few wild plants that were gathered during summer. Processed foods simply didn't exist, or if they did, they were minor components of their diet. As these people altered their native diet and became more and more westernized, their health began to decline, as Dr. Schaefer extensively documented in the medical literature of the time. Here's what Dr. Schaefer had to say about acne in 1971:

> *"Another condition has become prevalent, one obvious even to the layman: acne vulgaris. The condition used to be unknown among Eskimos, but one can see it readily amongst teenagers on the streets of Inuvik, Frobisher Bay, and Cambridge Bay. It is far less prevalent in the smaller centers. Old North men, such as missionaries, traders, trappers, men of the Royal Canadian Mounted Police and others who have known and watched the Eskimos closely for many years, frequently remark to their physician friends on the change in the complexions of the young people. Many Eskimos themselves blame their pimples on the pop, chocolate, and candies the youngsters consume as if addicted. One wonders what these people and the other old Northerners would think if they*

were to read some recent medical publications in which dermatolo-
gists belittle or deny the role of dietary factors in the pathogenesis
of acne vulgaris."

SCANT EVIDENCE

After having read this paper, I began to think that the real "myth" may have been the notion that diet had nothing to do with acne. One of my first stopping points was the position in the current dermatology textbooks. What was this information based upon? You might think that there was a long and well established trail of scientific literature conclusively demonstrating that diet and acne were unrelated, and that the remarks in the textbooks simply reflected well know facts. Nothing could be further from the truth! The viewpoint penned in these textbooks relied upon only two scientific studies of diet and acne that are now more than 30 years old. But more importantly, both of these dated studies contained fatal flaws in their experimental design which rendered their conclusions (that diet does not cause acne) erroneous.

Here's a case in point. In the often cited study by Dr. Fulton and colleagues (1969), examining the effect of chocolate consumption upon the development of acne, the authors gave the subjects a placebo (control) candy bar with a sugar content nearly as high as the chocolate bar. If sugar consumption has anything whatsoever to do with causing zits, then the experiment could never isolate this effect, since the treatment and control bars had nearly identical sugar contents.

Until late in 2005, the last dietary intervention concerning acne was published 34 years ago by Dr. Anderson. If the study by Dr. Fulton and colleagues was fatally flawed, then the study by Dr. Anderson was a complete joke! The subjects' baseline diet was not measured, so there is no way of knowing if the treatment diet differed from the subjects' normal diet. No control group was employed in the experiment, and the data (zit count) were not statistically analyzed, nor was the lesion (zit) count even presented!

Despite the shortcomings of these diet/acne studies from the late 1960's and early 1970's, there is information from an older era that points toward a link between diet and acne. Although these early physicians and dermatologists did not have the advantage of knowing the hormonal, biochemical and molecular underpinnings of acne, they were astute clinicians who carefully examined their patients and recorded detailed patient histories. In the 1920's and 1930's it was not uncommon for physicians to not only make house calls, but to spend an hour or more examining their patients to determine everything they could about lifestyles, environment and diet. After decades of practice, and having examined tens of thousands of patients, these physicians were able to formulate (admittedly non-scientific) informed hypotheses about the causes of acne. Check out this quote from "Taylor's Practice of Medicine 15th Edition" published in 1936 regarding the role of diet and acne:

> *"The internal treatment of acne vulgaris must depend*
> *on the symptoms presented by each individual patient. . .*
> *As regards the diet, it is usually important to restrict*
> *the amount of carbohydrate and fat, and sweets, cakes,*
> *pastries, puddings, jam and marmalade, pig-fat, chocolate . . .*
> *Plenty of fresh fruits and green vegetables and lean meat, fish*
> *and poultry should be taken."*

As you will see in later chapters most of this nearly 70 year old advice is right on target. However, 70 years later it can now be supported from clinical dietary trials that have shown how sugary foods and high glycemic load carbohydrates like those listed above can adversely influence the hormones that are directly involved in causing acne. The recommendation to eat fresh fruits, green vegetables, lean meat, fish and poultry now makes perfect sense with our new understanding of how diet can influence the hormonal, cellular and molecular underpinnings of acne.

THE TIP OFF

As you can see, the case against the causal link between diet and acne is weak, or non-existent. However, of more importance is the flip side of the coin: how do we know that diet is indeed responsible for acne? In science we use four procedures to establish cause and effect between diet and disease. Figure 1.1 below shows you these four procedures.

Figure 1.1. The Four Procedures to Establish Cause and Effect between Diet and Disease.

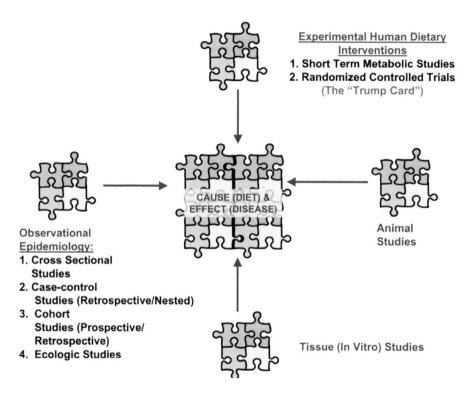

Experimental Human Dietary Interventions
1. Short Term Metabolic Studies
2. Randomized Controlled Trials
(The "Trump Card")

CAUSE (DIET) & EFFECT (DISEASE)

Observational Epidemiology:
1. Cross Sectional Studies
2. Case-control Studies (Retrospective/Nested)
3. Cohort Studies (Prospective/Retrospective)
4. Ecologic Studies

Animal Studies

Tissue (In Vitro) Studies

In the case of simple diseases like dental cavities, cause and effect are relatively easy to establish, because all four lines of evidence (epidemiological studies, tissue studies, animal studies and human dietary interventions) point in the same direction. With more complex diseases like coronary heart disease (CHD) causality is more difficult to establish because there are so many environmental and genetic factors that operate together to cause the disease.

Frequently, the animal studies may say one thing and the epidemiological studies may say another. When this happens, the results from human dietary interventions represent the trump card, and their results prevail. Human dietary interventions are the most powerful type of experiments because they can actually determine if a certain element of diet is responsible for eliciting a disease or disease symptom. For instance, if we eliminate vitamin C from a person's diet, they get scurvy. If we put vitamin C back into their diet, scurvy is cured.

THE EVIDENCE

Until late in 2005, the last dietary intervention involving diet and acne was conducted 34 years ago. Only two modern epidemiological studies (2002 and 2005) exist which have examined the relationship between diet and acne. However, having said this, there are literally thousands of dietary studies which indirectly link diet to acne via nutritional mechanisms. I have pointed out many of these relationships in my 2005 paper entitled "Implications for the Role of Diet in Acne" which you can download at my website: www.thepaleodiet.com

The first modern epidemiological study linking diet to acne comes from a paper my research group and I published in "The Archives of Dermatology" in 2002 in which we examined the incidence of acne in non-westernized populations. In the first part of the study my co-author Dr. Staffan Lindeberg from Lund University in Sweden examined 1,200 Kitavan people living on the remote Trobriand Islands off the coast of Papua New Guinea. The sample included 300 subjects who were between 15 and 25 years of age. Dr. Lindeberg and his co-workers did not find a single case of acne in the entire population including 300 teenagers and young adults. The picture you see below is that of an adolescent Kitavan girl with a representative acne-free complexion.

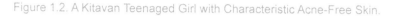

Figure 1.2. A Kitavan Teenaged Girl with Characteristic Acne-Free Skin.

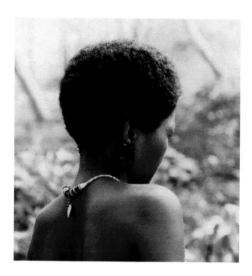

If you were to round up 300 teenagers in the U.S., Australia or the U.K., it would be virtually impossible to get a random group of 300 teenagers that were free of acne. Acne runs rampant in western adolescent populations. In fact, between 79-95% of all U.S. teens between 16 and 18 years of age have acne.

In the second part of our study my colleagues Drs. Kim Hill and Dr. Magdalena Hurtado examined 115 Ache hunter gatherers who were living in a remote jungle area in Paraguay. In this study we did things a little differently. We followed these people for more than 2 years and periodically examined them for acne symptoms. Once again, we did not find a single case of acne in the entire population, including 15 teens and young adults. The photograph you see directly below on this page is that of an Ache teenaged girl with representative acne-free skin.

Figure 1.3. An Ache Teenaged Girl with Characteristic Acne-Free Skin.

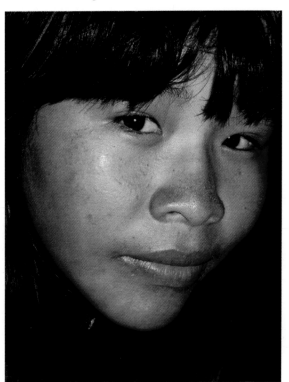

When we examined the diets of both the Kitavans and the Ache, they were quite unlike anything the typical U.S. citizen would normally eat. The dietary staples for the Kitavans were tubers (taro, yams and sweet potatoes), fruit (banana, papayas, mangoes, guavas and pineapples), fish and coconuts. Their intake of dairy, alcohol, coffee, and tea was nil, and their consumption of cereals, sugar, salt, vegetable oils, margarine, and processed foods was negligible or non-existent. Virtually all carbohydrate came from low glycemic load tubers, fruits and vegetables.

Similarly, the consumption of western processed foods by the Ache represented less than 10% of their caloric intake, whereas the bulk of their food came from low glycemic load carbs like manioc root and gathered wild plant foods. Twenty percent of their daily energy came from hunted, wild game and domestic meats.

Now let's contrast this to the typical U.S. diet (Figure 1.4 below), in which more than 70% of the daily calories comes from foods (refined sugars, refined and whole grains, refined vegetable oils, and dairy products) which the Kitavan and Ache people rarely ate. Later on in the book, I will explain to you precisely how all of these foods contribute to the development of acne by directly influencing the hormonal dysfunction that underlies acne and by displacing more healthful fresh fruits, vegetables, lean meats and seafood.

Figure 1.4. Energy Provided by Food Groups in the U.S. Food Supply.

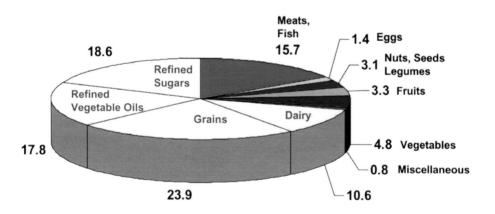

Refined sugars, grains, vegetable oils and dairy = 70.9% of energy in the U.S. food supply

Our paper was the first line of evidence to show from an epidemiological perspective that acne almost certainly was caused by an interaction of an environmental factor (diet) with genetic factors. How did we know this? When we looked at previous studies of South American Indians (with an overall genetic makeup similar to the Ache), those living in more westernized towns and cities had intermediate levels of acne – not as high as westerners, but certainly not absent as we reported in the Ache. Similarly, South Pacific islanders living in more westernized ways had a considerably higher incidence of acne than the Kitavans who were completely free of this skin disorder.

In February of 2005, an epidemiological study by the well known research group from the Harvard School of Public Health demonstrated that milk consumption was associated with the development of acne in a group of 47,355 women who had participated in the on-going Nurses Health Study. Although the authors of this study speculated that it may have been hormones from cow's milk that were responsible for this statistical association, I will show you later that a more likely mechanism was the high insulin response elicited by milk drinking as well as by milk's ability to impair zinc absorption.

THE TRUMP CARD

In November of 2005 I had the opportunity to address the Australian Nutrition Society in Melbourne and met up with my colleague and co-author, Dr. Neil Mann from the Royal Melbourne Institute of Technology. Neil had read our 2002 paper in The Archives of Dermatology and was familiar with my ideas of how the typical western diet could cause acne. He was fortunate to get funding to initiate an experimental study to test my hypotheses and in May of 2003 began a 2 and a half year dietary intervention in 43 acne patients. When I saw Neil in November of 2005 at the Nutrition Society meeting, he released the results of his study to the world. Diet, indeed, caused acne, and Neil and his co-workers were able to show how a high protein, low glycemic load diet improved acne symptoms as well as the hormonal problems that underlie acne. We finally had our trump card! We didn't have all the answers, but Neil's work represented the beginning – a ripple if you will, that will soon become a tidal wave that will re-write the textbooks of dermatology.

It will take a decade or more of research to precisely pinpoint all of the physiological and biochemical mechanism underlying the dietary links to acne. But you know what? You won't have to wait that long. You can begin to clear up your acne today by following the diet I prescribe. This is the diet that I recommend to not only clear up your acne, but also to maximize your health and normalize your body weight. It is actually not a diet at all, but rather a lifetime way of healthy eating!

THE BOTTOM LINE

• Although many dermatologists believe that diet does not cause acne, this perception is based upon only two flawed scientific studies now more than 30 years old.

• In 2002 my research group and I demonstrated that acne was completely absent in two non-westernized societies (The Kitavan Islanders living off the coast of New Guinea, and the Ache hunter gatherers of Paraguay) living and eating in their traditional manner.

• In the typical U.S. diet refined sugars, cereal grains, vegetable oils and dairy products comprise about 70% of the total daily caloric intake. Virtually, all of these foods were never or rarely consumed by either the Kitavans or the Ache people.

• In a just completed (2005) two and half year study of 43 acne patients from Melbourne Australia, a high protein, low glycemic load diet was shown to improve acne symptoms and the hormonal problems that underlie acne.

• You can begin to clear up your acne today by following the diet I prescribe. This is a diet that mimics the Kitavan and Ache diets with common, everyday foods available in the supermarket.

• The diet I recommend will not only clear up your acne, but will normalize your weight and maximize your health and well being. It is not a diet at all, but rather a lifetime way of healthy eating.

Success Stories

ACNE PATIENT TESTIMONIALS

The following 15 unsolicited success stories have been sent to me by acne patients, or their parents, from all over the world who have improved or completely cleared up their symptoms by following the dietary recommendations I provide in the chapters that follow. I list them in chronological order from most recent to earliest.

Teenaged Acne Sufferer in Australia... (Date: 6/13/05)

My name is Daniel (17 years old). I am an Australian resident currently suffering from mild acne. Over the past few months I have been studying and observing many articles on the Internet highlighting natural remedies for acne. I found that behavioral patterns and diet were key factors contributing to acne. My background is Middle Eastern, and a Middle Eastern diet is entirely centered on meals that involve bread. I would eat bread with everything-- breakfast, lunch and dinner involved bread. For a while now I have substantially reduced my bread intake and I have noticed an improvement in my acne. In mornings past, I would wake up and have breakouts, but that's reduced significantly. Today I decided to surf the net to find anything about acne that involved bread. I was AMAZED to find an article discussing your theory that eating bread and cereal may be a major cause of teenage acne. WOW. I just wanted to write and tell you you're doing a great job and I definitely think you are on the right path. I can't wait to hear more about your work. I have no doubt that research will only confirm what I've believed all along.

Thanks, Daniel

Another Acne Success through Diet... (Date: 5/19/05)

I saw that you were developing your studies in the acne link and thought I would share my story with you: I guess it began when I was about 12, my family had a history of bad skin, my brother did a course of accutane, my sister did antibiotics (which my younger brother is now on). I did not want to take this part so I searched for alternatives, mainly through diet. I did the vegetarian thing, then went vegan, then went 95% Raw for a year (in which my skin was actually at its worst!) I thought these diets where the way to heal my skin. About 8 months ago after 12 years of this I added in chicken and fish to my diet and then after reading your book adopted your diet. My skin was better from day one, it was clearer and I could see it starting to heal! I have had almost no breakouts during the past month (I notice a lack of sleep will bring them on, also I had a bowl of oats with whey powder the other day that resulted in 3 spots a few days later). I also stopped taking any supplements for that time. It is interesting to note that when I added back in a multi vitamin and a few oils (in soft gels) my skin was noticeably redder and this went away when I stopped taking the supplements. I am looking forward to the release of your next book in August and am very excited about the info it contains!

Kindest Regards,

Kristi

My Acne is Clearing... (Date: 1/18/05)

I wrote you an email about a year ago (I don't expect you to remember) about your published article on the diet-acne connection. You encouraged me to try your Paleo diet to control my acne. I've been eating the way you've outlined in your book and my face is amazingly clear. My only breakouts occur after a dietary slip-up (usually wheat or dairy). I've turned several other acne sufferers onto this way of eating and they've all seen drastic improvements. We really appreciate your work and the fact that your research goes "against the grain" (pardon the pun) of what dermatologists and others would ever say.

Thanks so much!!

Pete

No More Acne... (Date: 10/27/03)

I just wanted to take a couple minutes to thank you for information that has cured my 16 year struggle with acne. Since I was 11, I have had a moderate case of acne. It never was severe, but it has been very stubborn. I tried everything short of Accutane--several years of Retin-A, antibiotics, benzoyl peroxide, birth control, and every cream wash and mask available at the drugstore. I had the highest hopes for everything. I used Retin-A for about 4 years, thinking that one day it would magically kick in. Nothing ever worked. I was never without at least one major zit on my face, and I usually had several pretty obvious zits and lots of blackheads. Not fun, and definitely not psychologically helpful. Then I started doing research on the internet about the problem. I discovered your website and started reading the articles on it. I've always been a big carb fanatic--cereal for breakfast, lunch, and dinner was not uncommon. I decided to give the diet a try. I noticed that by the very next day, something felt different. I had no new eruptions. The ones I had started to shrink. After about a week, almost all my old zits were gone and no new ones took their place. I went on and off the diet several times until my experiments proved overwhelming. I now have been on the diet for awhile and have absolutely no breakouts on my face. And unlike the terrible side effects from my acne drugs (stomach problems, dry, itchy face), I have only the positive side effects of more energy, a clearer head, and a smile that I just can't shake. Plus the uncontrollable urge to go up to people at the grocery store and lecture them (but I'm too shy for that). The other thing I have noticed is that the growth of my little coarse chin hairs has slowed considerably. Maybe I'll get to stop tweezing them soon. An interesting thing happened last week at a conference. All of our food was already prepared and paid for, so I did cheat a bit. I didn't eat many carbs during the day, but at night I had quite a bit to drink (far too much, actually). The next morning my chin, where I have a tendency for breakouts, was swollen terribly with a boil, and I had 2 other zits on my face. My lymph nodes were also swollen. But after I got back on track, the boil is now completely gone with almost no mark. So again, I want to thank you. My whole attitude has changed, and I almost feel like a different person. Acne was very psychologically damaging to me, and the turnaround has helped so much more than just my skin. I just somehow wish all that money I threw down the garbage on the various acne treatments could have somehow gone to you instead!

Thank you,

Michelle

No Bread, No Acne... (Date: 9/18/03)

I read an article on the BBC website in Britain about your research into white bread being linked to acne. I myself have suffered from acne for a number of years and have recently cut bread out of my diet and I have noticed a big improvement.

Steven

Diet is a God-Send... (Date: 8/04/03)

I just thought I'd let you know. After reading your paper on acne and diet, specifically the affect modern diet has on insulin leading to acne... I have been strictly following your Paleo Diet in the book of the same name for more than a month now. I not only feel so much better, but after 10 years of hell my skin has stopped producing the excess oil it use to produce. This is a god-send. I can't tell you the relief this has brought to me. Thanks for writing the book.
Ash

My Face Looks Great... (Date: 5/19/03)

I live in Fort Collins, and came upon your article about acne. I'm 24 and have had moderate acne since high school. Accutane worked for awhile, less than a year, but then it came back... I was a serious cereal junkie too, cereal every meal every day. I got your book and follow your diet and I can't even tell you how much it's helped. My face looks great, I can't believe I didn't know this before; my dermatologist always said food had nothing to do with it. What an idiot.
Thank you so much,
Christina

Diet Helps Acne Patient... (Date: 4/13/03)

I am a 19 year old student living in New Zealand. I stumbled upon this website which reviewed an article that you wrote in the Archives of Dermatology. I would like to comment on your standpoint on the issue of acne in relation to diet. I doubt my viewpoint will be very useful to you as I have no medical background, but it may serve of interest. I suffer from PCOS and experience mild acne. I am currently on a course of Accutane. I have found that drastically changing my diet from the typical western diet of carbohydrates - sugar, junk, soft drinks, etc., virtually eliminated all forms of my acne. Upon stopping the diet and returning to unhealthy eating based around carbohydrates, my acne would return. I believe that there is a very important

17

link there. A diet high in carbohydrates such as sugar raises insulin, which elevates hormone levels, which contribute to acne. I have seen this in my own case. For years doctors have told women with PCOS to lose weight. Why? Because a loss of weight, a change of a diet high in sugar lowers insulin, lowers hormones, and thus drastically reduces acne. I do not know whether the same can be said for acne in males. I do believe that you are on to something. Keep doing what you are doing. All the best with your research.

Sincerely,

Monika

My Acne is virtually Gone... (Date: 4/08/03)

I would like to inform you that your recommendations you sent to me last week in regards to my question were put to good use and instant results were achieved. My acne is virtually gone!

Thank you again.

My Skin is Clear... (Date: 4/02/03)

I have consistently found that when I am on a low-carb diet, my skin is clear, but when I resume a "regular diet", I break out. My dermatologist and internist both looked at me like I was crazy when I shared this observation with them. It was very interesting to read about your study!

Robin

I Have Seen Massive Improvement... (Date: 3/07/03)

Dear Dr Cordain, I am writing to you regarding your article on Acne Vulgaris which was published in the archives of dermatology in December 2002. As a sufferer of acne myself at the age of 29 I was wondering whether it is the high glycaemic index of food or wheat allergy that is the cause of acne. Since your article was published I have gone on a wheat-free diet and I have seen massive improvement! In fact, I only got a spot in the last three months! I still wonder however, whether it is the wheat or the high glycaemic index. Have you done any trials on this? I would be grateful if you let me know what you have found.

Regards,

D. L., Ph.D.

Department of Molecular Pathogenesis, Institute of Neurology

His Spots Had Virtually Disappeared... (Date: 1/20/03)

My son Marc suffers (or suffered) badly from acne. He read with great interest a report on your research in New Scientist 17 December 2002. He immediately gave up all bread products and sugar. AT CHRISTMAS!!! At least we got to eat some of the sweets for a change! The effects were striking. His spots had virtually disappeared by Christmas day. Great joy! On the basis of this wholly unscientific experiment I can say that you seem to have identified the probable cause of his acne. The problem that we have is that he is determined to banish every last imperfection on his face. He is now extending his exclusions to all forms of carbohydrates. He has excluded all pasta and potatoes and is threatening to give up rice. The only form of carbohydrate that he will accept is muesli because the grains are still whole and will require some time to be digested. We are concerned that he must get some carbohydrates for his well being. I am sure that you have been bombarded with inquiries about your research but if you could give us some advice or direct us to your original paper we would be very grateful.

Roger

His Acne Improved Substantially ... (Date: 1/21/03)

Dear Dr. Cordain,

I was very interested in your paper concerning acne that you recently published and which received considerable media attention (Arch Dermatol 2002 138:1584-1590). Nutrition papers interest me in general because I am the assistant editor of "The Journal of Nutrition". Your paper interested me on a personal level, however. I have a son who is 18 y and who has struggled with acne for the last 3 years. He has tried various topical and oral products with limited success. He was ready to try Accutane but for several reasons I was opposed to this and have convinced him to try a low glycemic load diet instead. Interestingly, he consumed a gluten free diet for about 6 months beginning a year ago. I have celiac disease, as do several of my relatives, and he wanted to see if a gluten free diet improved his GI health and so he eliminated all sources of wheat, barley, rye and oats (due to possible wheat contamination). He was extremely strict about this diet and his acne improved substantially during this period. However, in addition to not eating gluten, his diet was generally better because he could not eat many processed foods, "normal" bread, etc. and so consumed more fruits, vegetables, home-made products etc. I would say he still consumed substantial carbohydrates because I make gluten free bread, cookies etc. and several commercial candy bars are gluten free. After about 6 months, he returned to a normal diet which rapidly deteriorated into a "standard" US teenage male diet. He did not notice any difference in terms of GI problems but gradually his complexion worsened and during the last couple months, the acne is worse than ever before. I was wondering if you have run across any papers relating acne to gluten or perhaps, wheat, or if most of the research concerns readily hydrolyzed carbohydrates in general. Are you planning to conduct any controlled studies of your hypothesis? If so, to how many grams of carbohydrate to you plan to restrict the treated group? I guess I'm asking for some guidance as I help my son test this treatment. (An n of 1 isn't a great experimental design but if it works, the single subject is going to be thrilled!!). I'll be watching eagerly for future papers from your group (Actually, this journal recently published one of your colleague's papers (Dr. Brand-Miller). Good luck with your studies and thanks for any additional information you can offer.

Sincerely,

K. H., Ph.D.

Assistant Editor

The Journal of Nutrition

My Acne Almost Cleared Up ... (Date: 12/01/02)

Dr. Cordain,

I just read the online Nature article entitled "Chips means zits". I want to share a couple of my recent experiences with you. First, some background. I'm 26 years old and I've had moderate/severe acne for over a decade. About 8 months ago I went on a low-carbohydrate diet and in addition to losing some weight (10 - 20lbs) I noticed that my acne ALMOST cleared up. Seeing my acne almost clear up in a matter of a few days and remaining almost cleared for several months afterwards fascinated me. Naturally I thought that the diet may have something to do with it. To test this hypothesis I went off the diet and in a week or so my acne came back in full force. I stayed off the diet for a couple of months and the moderate/severe acne continued as it has for much of my life. I then switched back to the low-carbohydrate diet and again, in only a few days, my acne almost cleared up. I'm currently wondering what will happen if I stay on this diet for a longer period than a few months will my acne clear up completely? That's what I'm planning on testing now. After conducting these experiments on myself, there is no question in my mind that a low-carbohydrate diet significantly improves my acne. And I suspect it will improve many other acne-sufferers' condition. Note that I have tried many medications and diets in the past in hopes of alleviating my acne and none of them worked (one exception is Accutane-though I had to discontinue it because of some negative side-effects). As a side-note, I've also noticed that my energy levels have increased significantly on the diet. On the diet I find that I'm more productive, more restless, and I require less sleep. The last side-effect I've noticed is a decreased ability to tolerate high-intensity exercise like running and weight lifting. In contrast, I seem to tolerate better lower intensity activities (e.g. hiking). I hope I haven't wasted your time.

Sincerely,

Evan

My Skin Has Improved Enormously ... (Date: 12/09/02)

Dear Professor Cordain

I was very interested to read your article this morning. I am now 52 years old - I had acne in my teens and have had 'spots' on and off ever since! I was eagerly awaiting the time when I would be too old for spots and too young for grey hair! - I have only succeeded in having a few grey hairs! However, in July of this year, I read an article in the Times about the basis of the 'Atkins' diet - i.e. cutting out carbohydrate. I had for years followed 'health advice' and had been eating a low fat high carbohydrate diet - the only visible effect of this was that I lost my lean shape, and put on inches round the hips. Since July, I have simply cut out, bread, potatoes, biscuits, cakes, pasta. Apart from losing five inches round my hips, my skin has improved enormously - what a bonus! Even before I read your article, I was convinced that my spots had not been the result of eating chocolate (eat very little of that) but that it was the other carbohydrates.

With kind regards
Penny
LONDON

THE BOTTOM LINE

- These wonderful success stories are clear-cut examples by people from all walks of life, and from all over the world, that demonstrate how simple changes in diet can improve or completely clear up acne symptoms.

- You too can join their ranks by following the dietary advice I offer in the following chapters.

- As opposed to every other dietary scheme involving diet and acne, my advice is based not upon opinion, anecdote or speculation, but upon firm scientific evidence – evidence that has now been substantiated by a newly completed dietary intervention of 43 acne patients from Australia.

- In the chapters that follow, I will show you precisely how some of the most common foods in your diet can cause you problems.

Acne Defined

MEDICAL DEFINITION OF ACNE

You know what they are – those bumps and spots on your face, your upper back, chest and elsewhere. Sometimes they become red, inflamed and infected. You call them zits, spots, pimples, blemishes, blackheads or whiteheads. They detract from your appearance, and probably cause you embarrassment and psychological discomfort. If your acne is severe enough, it can permanently scar your skin and change your appearance.

In medical jargon, zits, spots, pimples, blemishes, blackheads and whiteheads are all officially referred to as "comedones" (plural of comedo). It is interesting and perhaps somewhat ironic, from a dietary perspective, that in Latin, the word "comedo" means glutton. In the chapters that follow, I'll explain how over-consumption, particularly of certain foods, represents one of the major factors underlying the development of acne. Now let's get back to understanding what acne is all about.

THE ANATOMY OF A PIMPLE

Take a quick look at the Figure 3.1 on the next page. This is a cross sectional diagram of the pilosebaceous unit which is where all comedones arise. The central canal of the pilosebaceous unit is called the follicle, and its opening to the skin surface is called the pore. The follicle also contains a shaft of hair and an oil gland, known as the sebaceous gland. Even though pimples and blackheads frequently appear on your skin in places like your forehead where there seems to be no hair – there actually is hair. It's just that these hairs are so tiny and small that you can't easily see or feel them.

Figure 3.1. Cross Sectional View of the Pilosebaceous Unit which Consists of the Hair Shaft, the Sebaceous Gland, the Hair Follicle (Central Canal), and the Opening to the Follicle, the Pore.

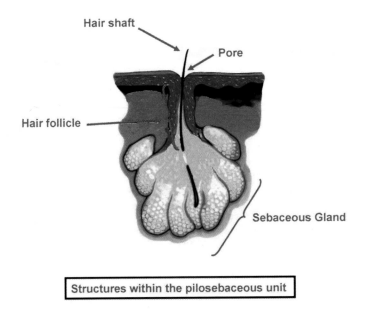

Structures within the pilosebaceous unit

TYPES OF PIMPLES

Comedones come in two basic forms: 1) closed comedones, or 2) open comedones. With open comedones, the pore remains open to the skin surface, but becomes enlarged and plugged with excessive skin oil called sebum and dead cells from inside the follicle. In lay terms, open comedones are usually called blackheads. In contrast, the pores of closed comedones become blocked to the outside skin surface by the cells that line the inside of the follicle. In lay terms, closed comedones are frequently called whiteheads. When whiteheads become enlarged or inflamed, you call them zits, spots or pimples. Both open and closed comedones can be classified according to their size and degree of inflammation. Table 3.1 lists the classification scheme that dermatologists use when describing open and closed comedones.

Table 3.1. Comedo Classification by Type, Size, Inflammation and Depth.

Comedo Type	Diameter
I. Open Comedones	1-5 mm
II. Closed Comedones	
1. Microcomedones	< 1mm
2. Closed comedones	1-2 mm
3. Closed macrocomedones	>2-5mm
4. Superficial inflammatory pustules	
5. Deeper inflammatory papules	< 5mm
6. Deep seated small nodules	5-10 mm
7. Deep seated large nodules or abscesses	>10 mm

Most acne patients have a mixture of non-inflammatory and inflammatory comedones, papules, pustules and nodules that can be classified into one of three levels of severity as listed in Table 3.2 on the next page.

WHO GETS ACNE ?

Most people think that acne is entirely a disease of adolescence and that after the teen years it just disappears. Not so! In the United States acne affects between 40-50 million people including young children, pre-teens, teenagers, young adults and even adults. Here are some of the numbers. In 10 to12 year old children, (28-61%) have clinically diagnosed acne, whereas (79-95%) of 16 to18 year old teens are afflicted.

Table 3.2. Gradation of Acne by Severity According to the International Consensus Conference Classification System.

Classification Description

Mild	Few to several comedones, papules, pustules, no nodules
Moderate	Several to many comedones, papules pustules and few to several nodules
Severe	Numerous comedones, papules, pustules and many nodules

It may surprise you, but a significant percentage of children (4-7 yrs.) are diagnosed with acne. In young adults over age 25, some degree of facial acne is found in 54% of women and 40% of men. Even older adults don't escape, as acne is present in 12% of middle-aged women and 3% of middle-aged men. And these numbers aren't just for the U.S. – similar values have been recorded in Australia and the U.K.

In the U.S. acne sufferers spend approximately 100 million dollars per year on over-the-counter treatments, and the cost to the economy from lost productivity, work absence and visits to physicians is estimated to be 1 billion dollars per year.

Now that you know all about what acne is and who has it, let's take a look at the fundamental causes of acne.

THE BOTTOM LINE

• In medical jargon, zits, spots, pimples, blemishes, blackheads and whiteheads are all officially referred to as "comedones" (plural of comedo).

• All comedones arise in a structure in your skin called the pilosebaceous unit.

• The central canal of the pilosebaceous unit is called the follicle, and its opening to the skin surface is called the pore. The follicle also contains a shaft of hair and an oil gland, known as the sebaceous gland.

• Comedones come in two basic forms: 1) open comedones, or 2) closed comedones.

• With open comedones, the pore remains open to the skin surface, but becomes enlarged and plugged with excessive skin oil called sebum and dead cells from inside the follicle. In lay terms, open comedones are usually called blackheads.

• With closed comedones, the pores become blocked to the outside skin surface by the cells that line the inside of the follicle. In lay terms, closed comedones are frequently called whiteheads.

• When whiteheads become enlarged or inflamed, you call them zits, spots or pimples.

• In the United States acne affects between 40-50 million people including young children, pre-teens, teenagers, young adults and even adults.

• In the United States, 79-95% of 16 to18 year old teens have acne.

4

The Immediate Causes
of Acne

ACNE: THE PROXIMATE CAUSES

The word "proximate" means immediate or nearby. The immediate causes of acne have been known for more than 40 years. In Figure 4.1 below, you can see that acne develops from four fundamental processes: 1) blockage of the follicle opening (pore), 2) excessive production of skin oil (sebum), 3) bacterial colonization and infection of the comedo (pimple), and 4) inflammation of the comedo and surrounding tissue.

Figure 4.1. The Proximate Causes of Acne.

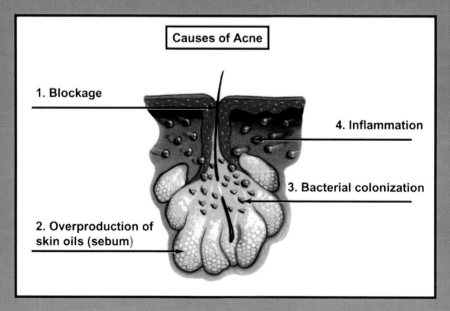

STEP #1: BLOCKAGE OF THE PORE

Let's take a closer look at step # 1 (the blockage of the follicle open-ing or pore) and see how the pore gets blocked in the first place. The cells that line the central canal (follicle) within the pilosebaceous unit fall into a category of cells in the body called "epithelial cells", a group of cells which may line either the inside or outside surface of organs and tissues. The epithelial cells lining the follicle come in two forms: 1) keratinocytes, and 2) corneocytes. Keratinocytes are formed at the basement membrane and move upward as they grow, mature and die in a process called differentiation. When keratinocytes die, they lose their cell nuclei and become flatter, tougher corneocytes which form the outside layer of your skin. Corneocytes are eventually shed in a process known as desquamation. It takes about four weeks for a newly produced keratinocyte to be shed as a dead corneocyte. In Figure 4.2 below you can see how these processes work when your skin is healthy and free from acne.

Figure 4.2. Normal Keratinocyte Differentiation and Corneocyte Desquamation.

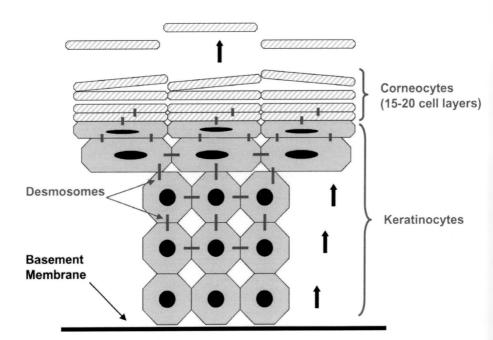

When you have acne, the opening of the follicle (the pore) becomes blocked by corneocytes that stick together forming rough scales. Additionally, this blockage is further fueled by excess production (proliferation) of keratinocytes which mature into scaly, rough corneocytes. In Figure 4.3 below, you can see how the pore becomes blocked by abnormal corneocytes. The reason why the corneocytes adhere to one another rather than sloughing off in the normal manner is because cell to cell connectors know as desmosomes remain intact during desquamation.

You can think about the entire differentiation and desquamation process as a life cycle. Keratinocytes are born, grow and die and then become corneocytes which form the 15-20 cell layers of your outside skin. Corneocytes move upward and are eventually shed during the desquamation process. Even though keratinocytes must die and become corneocytes which are shed to the outside, this process is healthy

Figure 4.3. Abnormal Keratinocyte Differentiation and Corneocyte Desquamation with Acne.

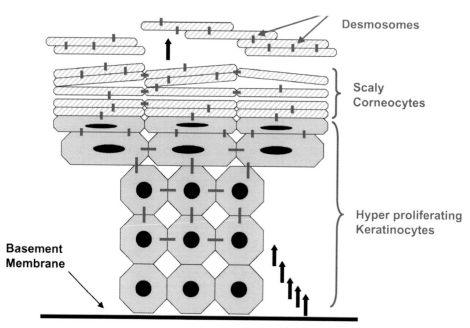

because it allows the body to continually replace older cells by newer cells and therefore rid itself of invading pathogens and damaged cells.

However, with acne, this life cycle of epithelial cells goes awry, and keratinocyte death occurs too late in the entire cycle. The scientific term for programmed cell death is "apoptosis", and with acne the delay in apoptosis is one reason why the desmosomes remain intact longer. I bring up this description of programmed cell death (apoptosis) not to complicate matters, but to show you an event that is crucial in understanding how diet represents the root cause of acne. Later I will show you how diet can adversely affect hormones which control apoptosis in the keratinocytes that line the follicle.

There also is a second reason why desmosomes remain intact. As keratinocytes begin to turn into corneocytes, the molecular structure of the desmosomes starts to change, and they begin to be composed almost entirely of three proteins called Dsg1, Dsc1 and corneodesmosin. In contrast, keratinocyte desmosomes may contain 10-15 different proteins. It is the failure of these three proteins within corneocyte desmosomes to decompose or breakdown properly that further causes the corneocytes to stick to together and block the pore. In the next chapter I will show you how substances in common everyday foods impair enzymes (substances that speed up chemical reactions) which are responsible for the disintegration of Dsg1, Dsc1 and corneodesmosin. This series of events represents one of the very first steps in the formation of the closed microcomedone (the tiny little pimple I described in Table 3.1).

I know that this all sounds a bit technical, but we need to get to this level so that you can understand how common, everyday foods can cause acne.

STEP #2: TOO MUCH SKIN OIL (SEBUM)

The second major proximate cause of acne is the overproduction of oil (sebum) by the sebaceous gland. The primary reason why these glands produce too much sebum is because they are being stimulated to do so by high levels of male hormones circulating in the blood stream. Your may not know it, but both men and women produce male hormones called androgens. In men, androgens are synthesized in the testicles, and in women they are made in the ovaries. The availability of androgens in the bloodstream is determined by a hormone produced in the liver called sex hormone binding globulin (SHBG). When blood levels of SHBG are low, the bioavailability of androgens in the blood is increased to all tissues. Conversely, when blood levels of SHBG are high, the availability of blood androgen to the body's tissues is low. Later on, I will show you how everyday foods, that you probably have been eating your entire life, can elevate the production of androgens from both the ovaries and testicles as well as suppress the liver's production of SHBG. The net effect of these diet-induced hormonal shifts will increase your blood levels of male hormones, which in turn will stimulate the sebaceous gland to produce excessive oil.

STEPS #3 AND 4: BACTERIAL INFECTION AND INFLAMMATION

Once the pilosebaceous unit is sealed over by overly adherent corneocytes, and once the sebaceous gland begins to produce too much oil, an ideal environment is now set up for bacterial colonization. *Propionibacterium acnes* is the name of a bacterium that normally lives without causing problems on the skin's surface. However, once the microcomedo (tiny zit) is formed, shutting off the follicle with its sebum rich environment to the outside air, the bacteria can now thrive inside the microcomedo. Certain substances found within the cell walls of the colonizing bacterium stimulate the immune system to produce localized pro-inflammatory hormones called cytokines. When the immune system gets revved up inside the pilosebaceous unit it can produce an inflamed comedo that we labeled a papule, pustule or nodule as previously defined in Table 3.1. This is what you know, all too well, as the red, fiery-hot, inflamed zit or pimple.

Remember that papules are the least serious of the inflammatory comedones, whereas nodules are the most serious. Over-production of inflammatory cytokines by the immune system underlies the development of the most serious nodular forms of acne. In the next chapter I will show you how diet can have a direct calming effect upon your immune system, and how certain elements of the typical western diet produce a net pro-inflammatory state which tends to promote the more serious types of acne lesions.

You now know the four proximate or immediate causes of acne, but don't you feel as if something has been left out? Isn't there something missing? What events ultimately trigger the four primary proximate causes of acne? This was the very same question I asked myself after having read Otto Schaefer's classical paper, so many years ago.

THE BOTTOM LINE

Acne develops from four fundamental processes:

1. Blockage of the follicle opening (pore) by cells called corneocytes that fail to shed in a normal manner

2. Excessive production of skin oil (sebum) caused by elevated blood concentrations of androgen hormones

3. Bacterial colonization and infection of the comedo (pimple)

4. Inflammation of the comedo and surrounding tissue

• These four mechanisms represent the "proximate" (nearby) known causes of acne.

• Of greater importance is the question, why do these four proximate causes of acne occur in the first place?

• In the next chapter, I fully explain how diet ultimately triggers the four proximate causes of acne.

5

The Ultimate Causes
of Acne

THE ULTIMATE CAUSES OF ACNE

O.K. – so now you have it! You are up to speed with your dermatologist. You know the four proximate or immediate causes of acne. But this knowledge really doesn't do you much good. You've still got your zits, and many dermatologists still won't acknowledge that diet has anything to do with your bad complexion. Do zits simply arise out of the ozone, or is there a scientifically based explanation for their appearance? Is this the Dark Ages or the 21st Century? Let's take a look at the facts – not as they were in 1971 when the last diet/acne trial was completed, but in the 21st century with 34 years of nutritional experiments under our belts.

Perhaps the most important question that scientists and physicians should be asking themselves in trying to figure out what factors ultimately cause acne is the question most often posed by children: the "Why" question. We know that overly adherent and scaly, rough corneocytes block the pore, but why do they become overly adherent to one another and scaly in the first place? We know that desmosomes remain intact causing corneocytes to become overly adherent and block the pore, but why do desmosomes remain intact in the first place? We know that there is an over production of keratinocytes (hyperproliferation) which eventually become corneocytes, but why is there a hyperproliferation of keratinocytes in the first place? We know that excessive androgens in the bloodstream stimulate the sebaceous glands to produce too much oil, but why are there excessive androgens in the bloodstream in the first place? We know that too little SHBG in the blood increases the availability of androgens to the sebaceous glands, but why is there too little SHBG in the first place? We know that an excessive immune response can lead to more severe forms of acne, but why is there an excessive immune response in the first place?

When we answer all of these why questions correctly we will be standing before the Holy Grail of dermatology – the ultimate cause of acne. Let's take a look at how diet is intimately involved in causing the known, proximate causes of acne.

The Glycemic Index

Before I show you how diet can cause the follicle to become blocked, I've got to bring up a concept called the glycemic index (GI). The glycemic index, was originally developed in 1981 and compares how various foods cause your blood sugar (glucose) levels to rise based upon equal amounts of carbohydrate in the food. In 1997, the concept of glycemic load (glycemic index multiplied by the carbohydrate content per serving size) was introduced to assess the blood glucose raising potential of a food based upon both the quality and quantity of dietary carbohydrate. Table 5.1 on the next page lists the glycemic indices and loads of various foods and shows you that refined grains and sugars nearly always maintain much higher glycemic loads than unprocessed fruits and vegetables. You can determine the glycemic index and load of almost any food by visiting my colleague and co-author, Jennie Brand-Miller's website: http://www.glycemicindex.com/. Jennie co-authored the "International Table of Glycemic Index and Load Values".

The importance of the glycemic index and load relative to acne is that they influence the release of insulin into the bloodstream by the pancreas. Foods made with refined grains and sugars (basically almost

Table 5.1. Glycemic Indices and Glycemic Loads of Various Food Groups. Glycemic Load = (Glycemic Index x Carbohydrate Content in 100 g Portions

	Glycemic Index	Glycemic Load		Glycemic Index	Glycemic Load
Grain Products			**Vegetables**		
Rice Krispie cereal	82	72.0	Baked Potato	85	21.4
Cornflakes	81	70.1	Sweet Potato	61	14.8
Rice cakes	78	63.6	Yam	37	8.4
Shred Wheat cereal	75	62.0	Rutabega	72	6.3
Graham wafers	74	56.8	Beets	64	6.3
Cheerio cereal	74	54.2	Carrots	47	4.7
Rye crisp bread	64	52.6			
Vanilla wafers	77	49.7	**Fruits**		
Stoned Wheat thins	67	41.9	Banana	52	11.9
Corn chips	63	39.9	Grapes	46	8.2
Muesli bar	61	39.3	Kiwi fruit	53	7.5
Bagel	72	38.4	Pineapple	59	7.3
Doughnuts	76	37.8	Apple	38	5.8
White Bread	70	34.7	Pear	38	5.7
Whole Wheat bread	71	32.7	Watermelon	72	5.2
All Bran cereal	42	32.5	Orange	42	5.0
Sugar / Sweets			**Dairy foods**		
Jelly beans	78	72.6	Ice Cream	61	14.4
Lifesavers	70	67.9	Yogurt, low fat	27	5.3
Table sugar	65	64.9	Skim milk	32	1.6
Mars bar	65	40.4	Whole Milk	27	1.3

all processed foods) elevate blood insulin concentrations whereas lean meats, seafood and fresh fruits and vegetables cause a minimal rise in blood insulin. Generally, the glycemic (blood glucose) response to a food and the insulin response are closely related. However, an exception to this general rule is dairy products, which have low glycemic indices and loads, but paradoxically cause high insulin responses similar to white bread. So, milk and cookies would not be a very good combination if you are trying to curb your body's insulin response.

If you are like the typical U.S. citizen, you have been eating highly glycemic and insulin stimulating foods your entire life. These foods comprise nearly half (47.7%) of the calories in the U.S. diet. See from Figure 5.1 below.

Figure 5.1. Per Capita Percentages of Highly Glycemic and Highly Insulinemic Foods in the U.S. Diet (1990-99).

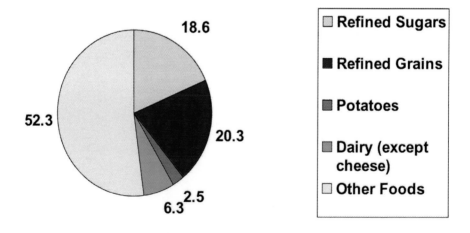

When you eat high glycemic foods, they keep your blood insulin concentrations elevated all day long, as you can see from Figure 5.2 below. This is not a good thing for acne sufferers, as I will shortly explain.

Figure 5.2. Day-Long Levels Of Insulin In 7 Healthy Male Subjects after three Days of Feeding Either High Glycemic Index (GI) or Low GI Meals and Snacks. Adapted from Kiens and Richter Am J Clin Nutr 1996; 63:47.

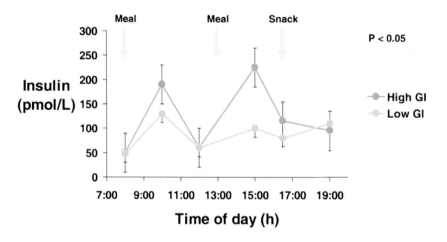

STEP #1: HOW DIET INFLUENCES BLOCKAGE OF THE FOLLICLE

Insulin Like Growth Factor Binding Protein -3 (IGFBP-3)

You now have the background to understand how the glycemic load works and how highly glycemic foods adversely influence your blood insulin levels. From Chapter 4, you know that one of the very first steps involved in the formation of the closed comedo is the blockage of the follicle by overly adherent corneocytes that form rough scales. You also know that corneocytes become overly cohesive to one another because there is a delay in, or impairment of, apoptosis (programmed cell death) in keratinocytes that prevents the desmosomes from disintegrating at the proper time. One of the most important hormones in the body that influences apoptosis is called IGFBP-3 (insulin like growth factor binding protein 3). Higher blood concentrations of IGFBP-3 accelerate apoptosis, whereas lower levels inhibit apoptosis. So, in order for the keratinocytes to get their timing right and die on time, the blood concentration of IGFBP-3 needs to fall into the right range.

Insulin is a master hormone and what it does influences almost all other hormones in the body, either directly or indirectly. High levels of insulin will reduce circulating levels of IGFBP-3, so when you eat high glycemic load carbs all day long, your blood concentrations of IGFBP-3 are going to fall, thereby delaying apoptosis in the keratinocytes lining the follicle. The delay in apoptosis partially prevents the desmosomes from fully disintegrating.

INSULIN LIKE GROWTH FACTOR 1 (IGF-1)

But there is more to it than just IGFBP-3 when it comes to hormones that can influence mechanisms that can block the pore. Once again, because insulin is a master hormone, it also affects another hormone called free IGF-1 (insulin like growth factor 1) which also is involved in the process that forms closed comedones. For virtually all cells in the body, free IGF-1 is a potent stimulator of cell growth and proliferation (formation). High levels of insulin in your bloodstream can cause blood levels of free IGF-1 to rise. Remember from Chapter 4 that the overly adherent corneocytes that ultimately block the pore develop from excessively proliferating keratinocytes deeper down in the epithelial cells lining the follicle. So, high glycemic load carbs elevate insulin. Insulin in turn elevates free IGF-1. Free IGF-1 may stimulate the overproduction of keratinocytes, which eventually develop into the corneocytes, which eventually block the opening of the follicle. I will shortly show you how other dietary elements also promote excessive keratinocyte proliferation.

One final note on the IGF-1/ IGFBP-3 story: hormones do not

act singly but rather like a symphony orchestra in which we hear the sum total of all instruments. IGF-1 and IGFBP-3 can bind one another at the surface of cells. When they do this, it impairs the action of IGFBP-3, which normally promotes apoptosis or cell death. When keratinocytes don't die on time, it promotes acne. So the binding of IGF-1 to IGFBP-3 is not a good thing for acne sufferers because as with high glycemic load carbs, it, in effect, reduces IGFBP-3.

Dietary elements are known to promote IGF-1 to IGFBP-3 binding. IGF-1 and IGFBP-3 are more likely to bind one another when high concentrations of a substance called "transglutaminase" appear at cell surfaces. In certain people, consumption of wheat or any food made from wheat can cause increased transglutaminase to be produced by various cells throughout the body.

So, high glycemic load foods composed of refined grains made from wheat, may do double damage – they reduce IGFBP-3 production in the liver from their high glycemic load, and they impair IGFBP-3's utilization within cells by increasing the likelihood of it binding to IGF-1 rather than to keratinocytes.

Interleukin 1 alpha (IL-1 alpha)

We're not quite finished yet with how diet can influence cellular processes that block the outlet to the follicle. You already know that overly adherent corneocytes (via intact desmosomes) are involved in the blockade of the follicle, but another factor contributes as well. It is the structure of the corneocytes themselves. With acne, as you can see in Figure 4.2, from the previous chapter, the adherent corneocytes form rough scales and adversely affect the final stages of desquamation, and therefore play a key role in blocking the opening of the follicle.

IL-1 alpha is a cell-to-cell messenger produced by white blood cells called monocytes. Because it is a localized hormone, it is labeled a "cytokine", and is one of a series of cytokines produced by white blood cells that are involved in pro-inflammatory processes. Scientists frequently can get at mechanisms of disease by isolating certain tissues outside the body in experiments called "in vitro" studies. In vitro experiments of isolated follicles have shown that added IL-1 alpha caused the follicle to form scales similar to what is seen in living acne patients. Additionally, comedones from acne patients have elevated concentrations of IL-1 alpha.

OK. So, let's get back to the "Why" question one more time. Why are follicular tissue levels of IL-1 alpha elevated in acne patients in the first place, and what dietary elements are known to lower IL-1 alpha? Before, we can get to these issues, I've got to do a little back tracking and give you a crash course on dietary fats.

Dietary Fats: The Basics

There are three basic categories of fats: 1) saturated fats, like what you find in butter, fatty meats and cheeses, 2) monounsaturated fats, like what you find in nuts, avocadoes and olive oil, and 3) polyunsaturated fats, like what you find in salad and vegetable oils. Virtually all real world foods that you eat are mixtures of these basic types of fat. So even though you may think of bacon as pure saturated fat, it actually consists of 66% saturated fats, 30% monounsaturated fats and 4% polyunsaturated fats.

In order to understand how diet can have a huge effect upon your immune system's inflammatory response, we need to take a closer look at the polyunsaturated fats which are divided into two sub-families: 1) the omega-6 polyunsaturated fats, and 2) the omega-3 polyunsaturated fats. In the typical western diet we have way too many omega-6 fats and too few omega-3 fats. In fact, most Americans eat 10 times more omega-6 fats as they do omega-3 fats. In non-westernized societies that are free of acne the ratio of omega-6 to omega-3 fats is about 2:1. It is this 10:1 imbalance between omega-6 and omega-3 fats in the western diet that is responsible for producing a constant pro-inflammatory profile in many of the body's tissues, particularly the white blood cells.

Omega-3 Fats, IL-1 alpha and Blockage of the Follicle

You now know that higher concentrations of IL-1 alpha within the follicle can lead to corneocyte scaling and roughness which may contribute to the blockage of the follicle's opening (pore) to the outside skin. And, it is this blockage of the follicle that is fundamental to the development of the tiny little zit, the microcomedo that eventually can become a full blown, inflamed pimple. During the initial stages of the formation of the microcomedo, *Propionibacterium acnes* invades the follicle and causes an immune reaction from white blood cells called peripheral blood monocytes (PBM) which react to the presence of the bacterium in the follicle by secreting pro-inflammatory cytokines, including IL-1 alpha, the cytokine known to disrupt normal desquamation.

The severity of the immune response by blood monocytes to invading foreign substances is very much influenced by diet. Hundreds of experiments in human, animal and isolated tissue studies have demonstrated that excessive omega-6 fatty acids cause a potent pro-inflammatory response characterized by high concentrations of pro-inflammatory cytokines, including IL-1 alpha. The flip side of the coin is that supplemental intake of dietary omega-3 fatty acids can suppress excess IL-1 alpha production. In your body, you need just the right amount of both omega-6 and omega-3 fats. Not too much omega-6 and not too little omega-3. It is this proper tone – the proper relationship between both omega-3 and omega-6 fatty acids that will allow your body to produce a healthy immune response to invading bacteria.

Too Much Omega-6; Too Little Omega-3

You may remember from Figure 1.4 in Chapter 1 that 17% of the calories in the typical U.S. diet come from refined vegetable oil. These foods are the major sources of omega-6 fatty acids in our diet, and are the primary reason why the western diet causes a pro-inflammatory profile that adversely influences the cytokines involved in acne. Take a

Table 5.2. Fatty Acid Composition of Salad and Cooking Oils.
MUFA = Monounsaturated fats, PUFA = Polyunsaturated fats, SAT = Saturated fats.

	(Omega-6/Omega-3) Ratio	% MUFA	% PUFA	%SAT
Flaxseed oil	0.24	20.2	66.0	9.4
Canola oil	2.00	58.9	29.6	7.1
Walnut oil	5.08	22.8	63.3	9.1
Soybean oil	7.5	23.3	57.9	14.4
Wheat germ oil	7.9	15.1	61.7	18.8
Avocado oil	13.0	67.9	13.5	11.6
Olive oil	13.1	72.5	8.4	13.5
Rice bran oil	20.9	39.3	35.0	19.7
Corn oil	83.0	24.2	58.7	12.7
Sesame oil	137.2	39.7	41.7	14.2
Cottonseed oil	258.0	17.8	51.9	25.9
Sunflower oil	472.9	19.5	65.7	10.3
Poppy seed oil	No omega-3 fats	19.7	62.4	13.5
Hazel nut oil	No omega-3 fats	78.0	10.2	7.4
Peanut oil	No omega-3 fats	46.2	32.0	16.9
Coconut oil	No omega-3 fats	5.8	1.8	86.5
Palm oil	No omega-3 fats	11.4	1.6	81.5
Almond oil	No omega-3 fats	70.0	17.4	8.2
Apricot kernel oil	No omega-3 fats	60.0	29.3	6.3
Safflower oil	No omega-3 fats	14.4	74.6	6.2

look at Table 5.2 on the previous page and you can get a feel for how bad this dietary fatty acid situation actually is. Remember that you get most of these vegetable oils in processed foods, margarines, spreads, and cooking oils rather than the oils that you may add to your salads.

As I previously mentioned the average omega-6: omega-3 fatty acid balance in the U.S. diet is about 10:1 – way too much in favor of omega-6 fatty acids at the expense of omega-3 fatty acids. The ideal ratio is about 2:1, and you can see from Table 5.2 that except for canola oil, none of the commonly consumed vegetable oils are acceptable when it comes to calming the immune response that is central in promoting acne.

I would also like to point out to you that in the historical literature, nuts have been sometimes associated with acne flare ups. If you take a look at Table 5.3, you can see that the omega-6 to omega-3 profile for nuts is not much better than for refined vegetable oils, and if you do not get sufficient omega-3 fatty acids from other sources, such as salmon or other fatty fish, chances are your diet will produce a slight pro-inflammatory tone.

Table 5.3. Fatty Acid Composition of Nuts and Seeds. MUFA = monounsaturated fats, PUFA = polyunsaturated fats, SAT = saturated fats.

	(Omega-6/Omega-3) Ratio	% MUFA	% PUFA	%SAT
Walnuts	4.2	23.6	69.7	6.7
Macadamia nuts	6.3	81.6	1.9	16.5
Pecans	20.9	59.5	31.5	9.0
Pine nuts	31.6	39.7	44.3	16.0
Cashews	47.6	61.6	17.6	20.8
Pistachio	51.9	55.5	31.8	12.7
Sesame seeds	58.2	39.5	45.9	14.6
Hazel nuts (filberts)	90.0	78.7	13.6	7.7
Pumpkin seeds	114.4	32.5	47.6	19.9
Brazil nuts	377.9	36.2	38.3	25.5
Sunflower Seeds	472.9	20.0	69.0	11.0
Almonds	no omega-3 fats	66.6	25.3	8.1
Coconut	no omega-3 fats	4.4	1.3	94.3

Dietary Lectins

We're not quite done yet with our why questions. Why does the follicle get blocked in the first place? The final factors we need to consider are dietary substances called lectins. In medical terms, lectins are called "anti-nutrients" because they can cause adverse and sometimes damaging effects to the body when consumed. Lectins are complex molecules found in common plant foods and may be composed entirely of protein or of protein and carbohydrate. If they contain both proteins and carbohydrates, they are given the scientific term "glycoproteins". Lectins act like super glue in the body and can bind and potentially disrupt normal function in almost all of the cells in the body.

Lectins were first identified by their ability to cause red blood cells to clump or agglutinate. Hence, when naming lectins, the last word is almost always "agglutinin". Common dietary sources of lectins are wheat (wheat germ agglutinin or WGA), soybeans (soybean agglutinin or SBA), kidney beans (phytohemagglutinin or PHA), green peas (Pisum sitavum agglutinin or PSA), peanuts (peanut agglutinin or PNA) and virtually all other grains, beans and legumes.

Because of their specific molecular structure, most lectins are extremely resistant to the digestive processes that normally degrade protein molecules in the gut. Both grain and legume lectins are also not completely broken down by cooking. Consequently, lectins arrive fully intact in the small intestine where absorption of nutrients occurs. Most large protein molecules simply cannot get past the intestinal cell wall barrier and into the bloodstream, and if they do, certain elements in the immune system bind them and prevent them from getting into the bloodstream. So for decades, most scientists and nutrition experts simply assumed that when you ate small amounts of lectins in common foods such as wheat, beans and peanuts, the lectins passed out of the body in the feces and never made it into the bloodstream. That is, until someone actually got around to feeding dietary lectins to animals and humans to see what would happen.

Animal studies from Dr. Arpad Pustzai's laboratory at the Rowett Research Institute in Scotland have clearly shown that wheat (WGA) and kidney bean (PHA) lectins show up in the bloodstreams of laboratory animals shortly after they are consumed. Once in the bodies of these lab animals, these lectins are not harmless, but interact with and ultimately disturb many tissues and organs.

OK, these are only animal studies – how about humans? Can food lectins penetrate our defenses and get into the bloodstream where they can then be transported to all of the body's organs and tissues? Yes, this seems to be the case. At least two studies involving humans have shown that we are no different from common laboratory animals when it comes to absorbing dietary lectins.

The Human Evidence

Dr. Wang and colleagues at the University of Liverpool in the UK fed five healthy adult volunteers 200 g of roasted salted peanuts. An hour later, peanut lectin (PNA) was found in their bloodstream at peak concentrations. It took more than four hours for the PNA to be cleared from the bloodstreams of these subjects.

More recent studies of human cultured tissue have shown that wheat lectin (WGA) easily gets by the gut barrier and can enter into circulation by a so-called "back door" in intestinal cells, called the EGF receptor. Normally, the EGF receptor acts like a lock, and only specific keys (called ligands) built by the body's machinery can fit into this lock. But unfortunately for us, the lectin from whole wheat products (WGA) fits perfectly into the EFG receptor of intestinal cells. Once WGA binds the EGF receptor it is swiftly shuttled into the intestinal cell's interior where it can wreak havoc upon the cell's inner machinery or it may enter the lymph system which delivers it to the bloodstream where it can get into all cells in the body bearing the EGF receptor. Other lectins found in kidney beans (PHA), soybeans (SBA), and peanuts (PNA) also act like keys which fit into intestinal cell's EGF receptor and can follow this same route into the body.

How Dietary Lectins Promote Acne

As I mentioned before, some lectins, such as those found in grains and legumes are pretty nasty substances and have a substantial potential for disrupting normal cell and body function, providing they can get into the body in meaningful concentrations. Consequently, scientists have generally refrained from conducting experiments in humans because it was considered unethical to give people substances which may damage their health. Our knowledge of the deleterious health effects of lectins then comes almost entirely from animal and isolated tissue studies.

Let's now consider how dietary lectins have the potential to promote acne. As we have previously discussed, one of the first steps in the formation of a zit is blockage of the follicle by corneocytes which adhere to one another rather than separating normally during the desquamation (sloughing off) process. You also know that the reason why these corneocytes stick together is because their cell- to-cell anchors (the desmosomes) fail to disintegrate properly and on time. Let's take a closer look at the molecular structure of desmosomes in Figure 5.3 below.

Figure 5.3. Molecular Structure of a Desmosome Connecting Two Cells.

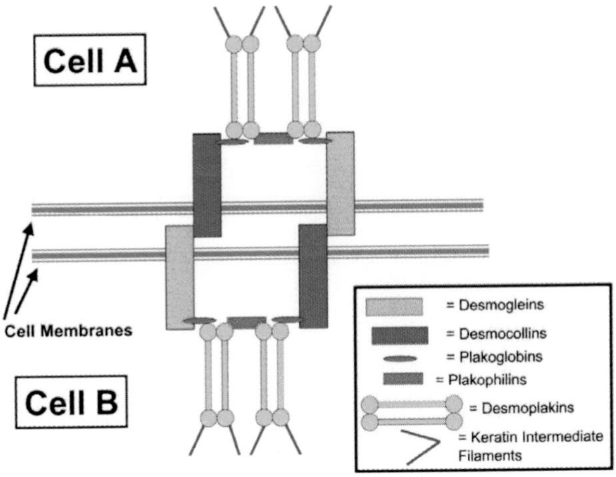

Figure 5.3 is pretty colorful and is made up of a whole bunch of molecules which are labeled in the key accompanying the diagram. But you really don't need to know a whole lot about this diagram except for two parts: the desmoglein molecules (colored in purple) and the desmocollin molecules (labeled in orange). These two molecules are half in and half out of adjacent cells. Their outside portions represent the cell-to-cell anchors that connect adjacent corneocytes. During normal desquamation, enzymes derived from underlying keratinocytes and from corneocyte structures, called lamellar bodies, dissolve the desmoglein and desmocollin molecules. It takes two kinds of enzymes to get this job done. First, carbohydrate dissolving enzymes, called glycosidases, and then protein dissolving enzymes, called proteases, must be applied. Proteases won't work by themselves, neither will glycosidases – both must be applied. The order is important also. To fully dissolve these two molecules, first glycosidases must be applied, then proteases. If one of these enzymes gets impaired then the corneocyte desmosomes will not disintegrate properly, and the corneocytes will stick together and block the follicle.

This is exactly what happens with acne. Common dietary lectins from whole wheat (WGA), peanuts (PNA) and soybeans (SBA) impair the action of one of the glycosidase enzymes, known as zinc alpha (2) glycoprotein or ZAG. This enzyme normally acts to dissolve three of the remaining proteins in corneocyte desmosomes: Dsg1, Dsc1 and corneodesmosin. However, when you eat lots of whole wheat, peanuts, soy based food products and other legumes, their respective lectins (WGA, PNA and SBA) get into keratinocytes and corneocyte lamellar bodies and bind zinc alpha (2) glycoprotein and prevent it from getting its job done. When ZAG can't get its job done and fails to completely dissolve Dsg1, Dsc1 and corneodesmosin, the corneocyte desmosomes remain partially intact, causing the corneocytes to adhere to one another. These overly cohesive and scaly corneocytes ultimately block the pore and represent one of the first steps in acne.

Other Effects of Dietary Lectins

Dietary lectins such as those found in everyday foods such as wheat, peanuts, soybeans and legumes are a double whammy for acne sufferers. They not only encourage cellular events which block the follicle by impairing ZAG, but they promote proliferation of basal keratinocytes. Remember that basal keratinocytes ultimately become the overly adherent corneocytes which block the pore.

ZAG is a multi purpose enzyme. It not only helps to dissolve the proteins that are found in corneocyte desmosomes, but it also slows keratinocyte proliferation, which is a good thing. If you are an acne sufferer you want to have reduced keratinocyte proliferation, and you want to have corneocyte desmosomes to dissolve normally. Any factor that prevents these actions promotes acne. When dietary lectins from wheat, peanuts, soy and legumes impair ZAG, they consequently prevent the normal breakdown of corneocyte desmosomes while also accelerating keratinocyte proliferation.

To add insult to injury, dietary lectins also promote the inflammatory processes that underlie the development of acne. I have previously shown you how increases in the inflammatory cytokine (IL-1 alpha), from imbalances in dietary fatty acids, promote follicle blockage. In additional to dietary fatty acid imbalances, numerous animal and tissue studies have also shown that WGA, PNA, SBA and PHA stimulate IL-1 alpha and many other pro-inflammatory cytokines and thereby contribute to follicle blockage via this mechanism.

Zinc Metabolism and Lectins

One further note on dietary lectins – the lectin from whole wheat (WGA) is potentially damaging to acne patients because it also impairs zinc metabolism. Once the WGA from whole wheat finds its way into cells via the EGF receptor as I have previously outlined, it directly blocks entry of cellular hormones into the nucleus of the cell. This spells disaster for zinc metabolism, as one of the most important zinc based proteins, metallothionein, is directly blocked entry into the nucleus by WGA. Zinc deficiency or inactivation of metallothionein has far reaching health effects including the production of pro-inflammatory cytokines by white blood cells. As an acne patient, your physician or dermatologist may frequently prescribe zinc supplementation to you because it is known to have a calming effect upon the inflammation that accompanies acne. But it's not just putting more zinc into your body to reduce inflammatory acne symptoms that counts – it's also improving zinc's uptake and utilization. By cutting down or eliminating the WGA from whole wheat, you will achieve this.

Dairy Products May Promote Acne

While we are on the topic of zinc metabolism, let me tie up a few loose ends. Your may remember from Chapter 1, the study from the Harvard School of Public Health that linked milk consumption to acne in a group of 47,355 nurses. The authors simply made a statistical relationship between milk consumption and acne, but did not actually determine why this relationship occurred. Milk may promote acne for two reasons. First, it is a concentrated source of calcium which severely impairs zinc absorption. Secondly, despite its low glycemic index, milk paradoxically has an extremely high insulin index similar to white bread. So, in regard to insulin metabolism, milk is no better than the refined carbohydrates which represent a primary dietary element causing acne.

STEP #2: HOW DIET CAUSES TOO MUCH SKIN OIL (SEBUM)

The second major proximate cause of acne is the over production of sebum (oil) by the sebaceous glands within the pilosebaceous unit. It is well established that excessive male hormones (androgens) in the bloodstream of both males and females can trigger the sebaceous gland to produce too much sebum. But the essential question is how do androgens get elevated in the first place?

Once again, to answer this question we must go back to foods that most of us have consumed almost every day of our lives – high glycemic load carbs. You know them. They are cookies, candies, breakfast cereals, chips, white bread, pizza, bagels, potatoes, white rice and almost all processed foods. Let's also not forget milk (whole, 2% and skimmed), yogurt, and sour milk. Besides impairing zinc absorption, which in turn may promote inflammation, these dairy products elevate your blood insulin concentrations just like high glycemic load carbs. High glycemic load carbs and dairy products set into play a hormonal cascade (elevated insulin, elevated IGF-1 and reduced SHBG) that causes increases in blood levels of androgens in both men and women. It is this increase in blood levels of the male hormone which directly causes the sebaceous glands to produce too much oil. Do yourself a favor, stay away from high glycemic load carbs. Your skin will thank you for it.

STEPS #3 AND 4: BACTERIAL INFECTION AND INFLAMMATION

We've pretty much taken care of the "why" questions for these two proximate causes of acne, but let's briefly summarize. The bacterium *(Propionibacterium acnes)* that invades the comedo requires an anaerobic (without oxygen) environment to colonize the comedo. If the pore didn't get blocked in the first place, the bacterium would remain on the skin's surface and wouldn't cause problems.

You realize by now that many dietary elements can act simultaneously to block the pore: 1) high glycemic load carbohydrates, 2) milk and other dairy products, 3) vegetable oils and 4) foods (grains and legumes primarily) containing dietary lectins. These are the same foods that promote inflammation. So we really can't separate the four ultimate causes (steps) of acne. Indeed, the symphony orchestra plays together, and almost all elements of the typical western diet contribute to acne at each of its four steps. As I pointed out in Chapter 1, the foods primarily responsible for acne (refined sugars, refined and whole grains, dairy products and refined vegetable oils) comprise 70.9% of the total food energy in the typical U.S. diet. Is it any wonder that almost every adolescent in the country has acne? Contrast these numbers to the Kitavan and Ache teenagers we examined who had no acne whatsoever, and ate virtually none of the foods that most of us eat on a daily basis.

Why Teens are More Prone to Acne

Did you ever wonder why teens are most susceptible to acne and why acne symptoms begin to subside as we age? Adolescence is a time of natural insulin resistance, and all people become more insulin resistant as they enter the teenage growth spurt years. Insulin is an anabolic hormone (meaning that it facilitates growth of all tissues). Because we are insulin resistant during our teen years, higher concentrations of insulin are present in our bloodstream, which in turn facilitates our adolescent growth spurt.

THE BOTTOM LINE

• The following commonly eaten foods promote acne: refined sugars, refined grains, refined vegetable oils, dairy products, whole grains and legumes.

• Refined grains, refined sugars and certain dairy foods keep your blood insulin concentrations elevated all day long and thereby cause a hormonal cascade that underlies the development of acne.

• When insulin is elevated, it lowers IGFBP-3, a beneficial hormone that promotes normal skin cell death (apoptosis) which prevents the pore from getting blocked.

• When insulin is elevated, it increases IGF-1, a hormone that stimulates excessive skin cell growth, and elevated IGF-1 prevents IGFBP-3 from doing its job.

• Refined vegetable oils contain too much omega 6 fats and too little omega-3 fats, thereby promoting excess inflammation through an inflammatory hormone called IL-1 alpha, which can cause skin cells to stick together and block the pore.

• Whole grains, beans and legumes contain substances called lectins which can get into the bloodstream and may promote acne by:

1. Inhibiting an enzyme (ZAG) that normally dissolves proteins holding skin cells together, thereby promoting blockage of the pore.

2. By inhibiting ZAG, lectins cause excessive skin cell growth which contributes to blockage of the pore.

3. Lectins increase IL-1 alpha and other inflammatory hormones.

4. Lectins impair normal zinc metabolism; low zinc concentrations in the bloodstream promote inflammation.

• Because of their high calcium concentrations, dairy products also impair zinc absorption and contribute to marginal zinc status.

• Refined sugars, refined grains and certain dairy products elevate insulin and IGF-1 which in turn cause the testes and ovaries to secrete too much androgen, a hormone which increases sebum production.

6

The Dietary Cure for Acne
Foods to Avoid

Let's get down to practical matters. You now know that diet is indeed responsible for acne, but what dietary items are you going to have to give up? Does this mean cutting out all of your favorite foods forever? Absolutely not, but you are going to have to make some major changes during the first 30 days if you want to get rid of your acne once and for all. Fall back too much into your old food habits, and your zits will return. Each and every one of us has a unique and slightly different genetic makeup. So it will be necessary to fine tune the diet to fit your specific food responses. Consequently, there are two phases to my dietary plan: 1) an initial one month (30 day) program in which you precisely follow the diet and 2) a more extended period lasting up to three months and beyond, during which time you add in single foods and see how your skin responds. If you get flare ups with these foods, then you will know that you will need to avoid them.

HOW LONG WILL IT TAKE?

Let me make it clear from the start. If you have suffered from acne for years and have had the severest form of acne that has caused scarring, no dietary treatment in the world will get rid of your scarring. However, even if you do have scarring, you can stop this disease dead in its tracks so that no future damage to your skin will occur. From Chapter 4, you may remember that it takes about a month for a newly formed basal keratinocyte to divide, grow, die, turn into a corneocyte and then be eventually shed at the surface of the skin. So, in most cases by strictly adhering to the diet for 30 days or slightly longer, you should experience dramatic improvement in your acne symptoms. Within days or a week of adopting the diet, much of the inflammatory symptoms of acne will begin to subside, because your new diet will be an anti-inflammatory diet.

PHASE 1: THE FIRST 30 DAYS

For the first 30 days of your diet, I recommend that you strictly (meaning as close to 100% compliance as is possible) follow the diet I have outlined in my previous book, "The Paleo Diet" (www.thepaleo-diet.com). Basically, this means eating only fresh fruits, vegetables, lean meats, fish and seafood. You will need to cut out all processed foods, both refined and whole cereals, refined sugars, legumes and dairy products. If the food comes in a can, a box, a bag, a bottle, a jar, or a carton, you will want to generally stay away from it. What you are after is fresh, living food – food that will spoil if it is not refrigerated and consumed within a few days or a week after its harvest. If you have ever paid any attention to how supermarkets are set up, you will know where to find these foods. The produce, meat and seafood sections of virtually every modern supermarket are located on the outside aisles, whereas the processed and junk food sections are found on the inside aisles. Perhaps the marketing and advertising experts are trying to subtly tell us something? Do we really need to march through the junk food aisles to get to the real food?

Foods to Avoid

Let's get down to the particulars of the diet. Table 6.1 includes a laundry list of foods that should be avoided for the first 30 days of the diet.

Table 6.1. Foods to Avoid.

Dairy Foods

1. Milk
2. Cheeses
3. Butter
4. Cream
5. Yogurt
6. Ice cream
7. Ice milk
8. Frozen yogurt
9. Powdered Milk
10. Non fat dairy creamer
11. Dairy spreads
12. All processed foods made with any dairy products
13. Sour milk, kumis

Cereal Grains

1. Wheat (bread, rolls, muffins, noodles, crackers, cookies, cake, doughnuts, pancakes, waffles, pasta, spaghetti, lasagna, wheat tortillas, pizza, pita bread, flat bread and all processed foods made with wheat or wheat flour)

2. Rye (Rye bread, rye crackers and all processed foods made with rye)

3. Barley (barley soup, barley bread, and all processed foods made with barley)

4. Oats (Quaker oats, rolled oats, and all processed foods made with oats)

5. Corn (corn on the cob, corn tortillas, corn starch, corn syrup, corn chips, Doritos, Fritos, Taco shells)

6. Rice (All rice, brown rice, white rice, top ramen, rice noodles, basmati rice, rice cakes, rice flour and all processed foods made with rice)

7. Wild Rice

8. Millet

9. Sorghum

10. Modified food starch (may be made from the grains: corn, wheat, or rice and from starchy tubers: potatoes, or tapioca)

Cereal Grain-Like Seeds

1. Amaranth

2. Quinoa

3. Buckwheat

Legumes

1. All beans (kidney, pinto, navy, white, lima, black, broad bean, tepary, wax beans, string beans, green beans, mung beans)

2. Lentils

3. Peas, split peas, snow peas

4. Peanuts (peanuts are a legume and not a nut)

5. Soybeans and all soybean products

6. Garbanzo beans, chickpea

7. Black eyed peas

Starchy Tubers

1. Potatoes

2. Cassava root, manioc

3. Tapioca pudding

Yeast Containing Foods

1. All baked goods (breads, doughnuts, rolls, muffins etc.)

2. All fermented foods (beer, wine, pickled foods, foods containing vinegar, tofu)

Fatty, Processed & Canned Meats & Fish

1. Sausages, bacon
2. Fatty hamburger
3. Fatty cuts of meats
    a. T-bone steaks
    b. Beef ribs
    c. Lamb roasts and chops
4. Processed meats
    a. Lunchmeat, deli meat
    b. Any preserved or smoked meat (hams, turkey, etc.)
    c. Smoked or dried and salted fish
5. Canned or pickled meat and fish
    a. Canned fish (tuna, sardines, herrings, smoked oysters and clams, canned salmon and mackerel, etc.)
    b. Canned hams, chickens, beef, etc.

Alcoholic beverages

1. All alcoholic beverages
    a. Note that these are permitted in moderation a number of days per week after the initial 30 period.

Sweets

1. All candy
2. All refined sugars
3. Maple sugar
4. Date sugar
5. Syrups
6. Honey
7. Dried fruit

Vegetable and Salad Oils, Margarines and Shortening

1. All processed foods made with or cooked in vegetable oils, margarines or shortening

2. The only exceptions are: flaxseed oil, canola oil, walnut oil and olive oil (see Table 5.2 in Chapter 5)

Initially, these suggestions seem like an enormous laundry list with seemingly needless removal of entire foods groups. But there is a method to this madness, as I have extensively documented in the previous chapters and in my scientific publications on diet and acne. When you adopt this diet, not only will your acne disappear, but your health will soar as well.

Rationale for Avoiding These Foods

In Chapter 5, I gave you the scientific details why certain foods in Table 6.1 may promote acne, either individually or in concert with other foods. Virtually all processed foods are made up of the same old 3 to 5 ingredients (refined grains, refined oils, refined sugars, dairy products, salt and perhaps artificial flavoring and coloring). These are the same foods that are instrumental in causing acne. Let me summarize why you should avoid the foods I have listed in Table 6.1.

1. Dairy Products

Except for butter, virtually all dairy products severely impair zinc absorption because of their high calcium concentrations, thereby leaving you at a greater risk for becoming zinc deficient. Zinc deficiency frequently occurs in acne patients and promotes one of the key elements underlying acne: inflammation. Your dermatologist may frequently prescribe zinc supplements to reduce the inflammatory symptoms of acne.

Whole milk, skim milk, yogurt, and sour milk despite having low glycemic responses, paradoxically elevate your blood insulin levels similar to eating a slice of white bread. Because these dairy products elevate insulin, they elicit a hormonal cascade similar to high glycemic load carbohydrates (increased insulin, increased IGF-1, reduced IGFBP-3). As I have pointed out in Chapter 4, this series of hormonal events promotes proliferation of keratinocytes and the abnormal desquamation of corneocytes, two of the key events underlying the blockage of the pore.

By elevating insulin, whole milk, skim milk, yogurt and sour milk will also elevate blood androgen (male hormone) concentrations and simultaneously suppress SHBG (the hormone secreted by the liver which normally lowers blood androgens). Elevated blood androgens directly stimulate excess oil production (sebum) which is one of the fundamental underlying causes of acne.

How about butter? It has virtually no calcium, so it will not impair zinc metabolism and by itself produces low blood glucose and insulin responses. So, in theory, it should not adversely affect acne. However, I would like to point out that butter is a high dietary source of saturated fat. This is the kind of fat that clogs your arteries and may predispose you to coronary heart disease. If you consume butter, consume it sparingly. A better choice for added or cooking fats would be olive oil which contains mainly heart-healthy monounsaturated fats.

2. Cereal Grains (Refined Grains)

From Table 5.1 in Chapter 5 you can see that virtually all refined grains, regardless of their physical form (breakfast cereals, cookies, chips, white bread, bagels, wafers, crackers, doughnuts etc.), have high glycemic indices and loads. Because of these characteristics they once again adversely affect insulin metabolism and cause a hormonal cascade (increased insulin, increased IGF-1, reduced IGFBP-3) which encourages the blockage of the pore.

Just like certain dairy foods, high glycemic load cereal grains also promote excessive oil production from the sebaceous gland because elevations in insulin and IGF-1 directly stimulate male hormone production in both men and women. Likewise, refined cereals suppress the liver's output of SHBG which normally helps to lower male hormones in the bloodstream. The net effect of regular consumption of high glycemic load cereals will be to increase androgen concentrations in the bloodstream which in turn will cause an overproduction of sebum (oil), which represents a key event causing acne.

High glycemic load carbohydrates also seem to worsen inflammation. There is a hormone that physicians' measure in your blood called C Reactive Protein (CRP). It is reflective of your net state of inflammation. High concentrations of CRP mean greater inflammation; lower concentrations mean less inflammation. A number of recent epidemiological studies have shown that high glycemic load carbs are associated with greater inflammation as measured by CRP. It should also be pointed out that the milling of refined grains removes approximately 80% of the zinc found in whole grains. So, consumption of refined grains may contribute to a reduced zinc intake. And once again, marginal or deficient zinc status may promote the inflammation characteristic of acne.

3. Cereal Grains (Whole Grains)

Whole grains are generally thought of by most physicians, nutritionists and lay people alike as wholesome, nutritious foods that promote good health and well being. However, there is a darker side to cereal grains that is infrequently brought up in the scientific or popular health literature. In their whole, unrefined state, cereal grains contain high concentrations of anti-nutrients. These are substances that may directly impair absorption of nutrients or worse still, interact with our bodies and produce adverse effects ranging from mild to toxic. There are six grains that we commonly consume in the western world (wheat, rye, barley, oats, corn, and rice) and all six contain a variety of anti-nutrients (lectins, protease inhibitors, alkylresorcinols, and alpha amylase inhibitors, among others).

The most extensively studied of these anti-nutrients is the lectin found in whole wheat called wheat germ agglutinin (WGA). One thousand grams of wheat germ that you buy in the grocery store contains between 300–450 mg of WGA, whereas whole wheat flour contains between 30-50mg of WGA per 1,000 grams of flour. As I mentioned in Chapter 5, it is now evident that WGA can enter the body through a special back door passage in the gut called the EGF- Receptor. Once in the body it can wreak havoc with many of our cellular enzyme systems that influence the development of acne.

First, regular consumption of whole wheat contributes to zinc deficiency. Most of the zinc in whole wheat is bound to an anti-nutrient called phytate which prevents its absorption in the small intestines. Secondly, WGA interferes with normal zinc metabolism in all epithelial and endothelial cells by blocking the entry of a key zinc substance called metallothionein into the nucleus. All of these events promote overall inflammation in the body. But worse still, WGA by itself stimulates white blood cells to produce localized pro-inflammatory hormones called cytokines. Inflammation is something you want to reduce if you have acne. Your dermatologist may prescribe a zinc supplement to help curb the body's inflammatory response. But a better strategy would be to get rid of the foods (like whole grains) that are impairing zinc absorption and utilization in the first place.

As I outlined in Chapter 5, WGA and other lectins from peanuts (PNA) and kidney beans (PHA) may work in concert with other dietary elements to block the pore by promoting keratinocyte proliferation and by impairing the normal desquamation (shedding) of corneocytes. Both of these processes represent one of the very first events that cause acne.

4. Cereal-like Seeds
Most of us have never tasted amaranth, quinoa or buckwheat. All three of these seeds are not technically grains because they are not

members of the grass family, of which all true grains belong. These pseudo grains are not much better than are traditional grains in that the bulk of their food energy comes from rapidly absorbable carbohydrate. For instance, buckwheat is 83% carbohydrate, quinoa 74% carbohydrate and amaranth 69% carbohydrate. Better food choices for your carbohydrates are fresh fruits and veggies.

5. Legumes

The story with legumes is very much the same as with whole grains. Remember that peanuts are really not nuts, but are rather a member of the same family (legumes) as beans, lentils and peas. Legumes impair zinc absorption because of their high phytate content and as such may contribute to zinc deficiency and ultimately promote inflammation. Virtually all legumes are concentrated sources of lectins and the lectins from peanuts (PNA) and kidney beans (PHA), navy beans (PHA, pinto beans (PHA), and string beans (PHA), rapidly (within an hour) enter the bloodstream after they are ingested. It is likely that these lectins enter the body through the same back door (the EGF receptor) that wheat lectin (WGA) does.

Like WGA, legume lectins directly cause white blood cells to produce localized inflammatory hormones called cytokines. They also can impair the ability of an enzyme (zinc alpha 2 glycoprotein) to regulate normal keratinocyte proliferation and corneocyte desquamation. Consequently, these legume lectins may be instrumental in blocking the pore, which again represents one of the key events in the formation of a pimple.

6. Starchy Tubers

Potatoes are far and away the most common starchy tuber that we eat. Because of their concentrated starch, they are high glycemic load carbohydrates that adversely affect insulin metabolism similar to re-fined cereal grains. Once again, the hormonal cascade caused by any food which spikes our blood glucose and insulin concentrations can promote acne through all of the avenues I have previously outlined. During the 30 day run-in of this diet, you should severely restrict your potato consumption in all forms. This means not only potato chips and French fries, but also baked and boiled potatoes.

Other starchy tubers that you may want to avoid during the initial 30 day run-in are sweet potatoes, yams and cassava roots. However, after your acne symptoms begin to subside these tubers frequently will not cause your acne to re-appear because they generally maintain low glycemic loads. As we get into the second step of the diet, I will fully explain how you can gradually re-introduce certain foods to determine if they cause problems.

7. Yeast Containing Foods

I include yeast containing foods on the avoidance list, not so much that there is any link between yeast itself and acne, but rather because these foods are almost always wheat or grain containing items such as baked goods. For some people with autoimmune diseases (diseases in which the body's immune system attacks its own tissues), there is some evidence to suggest that yeast containing foods may contribute to the disease process. Again, for the initial 30 day trial, try to avoid these foods. You can always experiment by adding them back in, once your acne symptoms improve or disappear.

8. Fatty, Processed & Canned Meats & Fish

Almost all of these foods will have little or no deleterious effect upon acne symptoms because they do not cause an unfavorable effect upon insulin metabolism. However, like butter, they tend to have high concentrations of saturated fat which can elevate your blood choles-terol levels and in adults increase your risk for cardiovascular disease. Use fatty, processed and canned meats and fish with caution. The fresh, leaner versions will always be a healthier choice, but water packed canned tuna or salmon are good second choices.

9. Alcoholic Beverages

For adolescents, this food category is not part of the legal picture, but if you are a young or even middle-aged adult suffering from acne, I suggest that you avoid alcohol for the 30 day run-in period, particularly beer, ale and other beverages manufactured from wheat, rice and barley. Also, sweet mixed drinks containing refined sugar need to be restricted. However, having said this, moderate alcohol consumption is known to improve insulin metabolism and in the long run may help to improve acne symptoms. If you enjoy an occasional drink, feel free to add these beverages back into your diet during the 2nd phase of the program and carefully monitor your symptoms, but avoid sweetened mixers like colas and tonic.

10. Sweets

All refined sugars have a great potential to adversely influence insulin metabolism and as such should be avoided for all of the reasons I have previously outlined. Refined sugars, like refined grains elicit hormonal changes that work together with other elements of the typical western diet to block the pore by promoting keratinocyte proliferation and abnormal corneocyte desquamation. Additionally, refined sugars are devoid of zinc and therefore contribute to a marginal or deficient zinc status, which in turn contributes to an increased inflammatory response that is characteristic of acne. In the U.S., 73% of the entire population does not achieve the daily recommended intake of zinc.

Finally, refined sugars set off a hormonal cascade that increases circulating male hormone concentrations which directly increase the amount of oil secreted by the sebaceous glands. Do yourself a favor and satisfy your sweet tooth with fresh fruit.

11. Vegetable and Salad Oils, Margarines and Shortening

If you are like the typical American, almost 18% of your daily calories come from refined vegetable oils, salad oils, margarine and shortening. We consume these artificially produced fats primarily from baked goods, processed foods and condiments. Check out a few food labels on almost any processed food and you will find some sort of vegetable oil as an ingredient. The big problem with vegetable oils, as I have already stated in Chapter 5, is that they contain way too much omega-6 fats at the expense of omega-3 fats. Take a look at Table 5.2 in Chapter 5 to get the numbers. The net result of our increased consumption of omega-6 fats at the expense of omega-3 fats results in a pro-inflammatory state which contributes not only to acne but also to heart disease, cancer and autoimmune diseases.

Because you will be avoiding almost all processed food and refined vegetable oils during your initial 30 day run-in diet, your consumption of omega-6 fatty acids will be severely curtailed, and your net inflammatory state will be nicely reduced, particularly if you include more fatty fish, a good source of omega-3 fats, in your diet. Increased consumption of omega-3 fats will not only decrease inflammation, it also will decrease blood concentrations of a cytokine (a localized hormone) called IL-1 alpha. The excessive presence of this cytokine in the blood is known to cause the abnormal desquamation and scaling that blocks the pore. Omega-3 fats are just plain good medicine for your skin.

PHASE 2: THE NEXT THREE MONTHS AND BEYOND

For the first 30 days of the diet, you will need to avoid, as best as you can, the foods I have listed in Table 6.1 of this Chapter. In the next Chapter I will show you the wonderful cornucopia of healthful foods that you may eat. Your taste buds and palette will be pleasantly surprised when you replace your processed foods made with the same old four ingredients (refined grains, refined oils, refined sugars, and salt) with delicious fresh fruits, vegetables, lean meat and seafood.

Moreover, your skin is going to love you for getting rid of processed foods. And you will like your new image along with increases in your energy, health and well being that most people notice as they adopt this lifetime program of eating. Check out the "Success Stories" icon at my website: www.thepaleodiet.com and see how others have succeeded in not only getting rid of their acne, but in improving their overall health.

Dialing In Your Individual Diet

Most of you will experience a gradual improvement in your acne symptoms within days to a week after adopting the dietary guidelines I have laid out. After 30 days or slightly longer, if you have been compliant with the diet, you should experience great improvements or complete remission of your acne. My advice is to remain on the strict run-in diet for as long as it takes to have a dramatic improvement or complete remission of your symptoms.

Once you have achieved clearance of your acne symptoms, you now may experiment with your diet to identify the foods that may be added back into your diet in limited quantities without causing problems. However, consumers beware! This is not a license to return to your old ways. The diet you have adopted is not a temporary plan to get rid of your zits and then go back to your normal diet. Your new program is a lifetime way of eating that will not only eliminate your acne, but will improve almost all other aspects of your health.

Taboo Foods: How Much, How Often?

One of the best ways to get somebody to not do something (not follow a diet) is to tell them they must completely and totally give up something they enjoy. All of us have favorite foods. Some people like chocolate, others ice cream, and some go for salsa and chips. Whatever your favorite food, it would be hard to even think about giving it up forever. Am I asking you to do this? – Absolutely not.

From a behavioral aspect, a little cheating may be good if it can keep you on the program. This is the approach that I take in keeping you on the diet that will improve or eliminate acne. If you eat three meals per day, then there are 21 meals a week and 84 meals a month. If you are 95% compliant with the diet, then this means that you may eat four "open" meals a month. By "open" meals, I mean you may eat whatever you please. If spaghetti and meatballs is your thing, go for it – don't eliminate it, but don't eat it regularly. I believe that many people can experience significant improvements in their acne symptoms by being only 90% compliant (eight open meals per month).

Adding Foods Back

The key to your long term success will be to listen to your body. Once you have cleared up your acne with the "strict" version of the diet, you should experiment over the next few months by adding in certain foods to see if they cause flare-ups. My advice is to only add in a single food or food type once a month. Give it some time and see if your symptoms worsen or stay the same. You may find that you can eat pizza once a week with no problems, but pizza 3 days in a row will cause problems. Similarly, you may find that some of the foods in Table 6.1 may have little or no effect upon your symptoms, such as legumes, sweet potatoes, tofu, pickled foods, vinegar or grated cheese on a salad. However, remember that the further you drift from the basics of the diet, the greater will be the chances of your acne returning. Try not to think of this as an "anti-acne diet", but rather a lifetime plan of eating that will improve your health and reduce your risks of getting the chronic diseases (heart disease, high blood cholesterol, hypertension, type 2 diabetes, cancer, autoimmune disorders) that afflict almost 70% of all adults in the U.S.

THE BOTTOM LINE

• Because it takes about 30 days or slightly longer for your skin cells to completely renew themselves, you will need to strictly adhere to the diet for about a month.

• Most people will experience improvement in their symptoms within a few days to a week.

• For the strict 30 day phase of the diet, the following foods need to be avoided: refined sugars, refined grains, refined oils, dairy products, legumes, whole grains, and potatoes. Since all processed foods are really nothing more than mixtures of sugars, grains, oils and dairy products, these foods should be avoided or eliminated for the 30 day run-in.

• After you have experienced dramatic improvement or complete elimination of your acne, then the second phase of the diet begins in which you gradually add certain foods back into your diet.

• Carefully monitor your symptoms as you add more and more food back into your diet

• Adding food back into your diet isn't a license to go back to your old way of eating. "The Dietary Cure for Acne" is not a diet at all but a brand new healthful way of eating for life.

7

The Dietary Cure for Acne
The Good Foods

WHAT YOU WILL BE MISSING BY ELIMINATING DAIRY AND GRAINS

Most party line nutritionists wouldn't object to my advice to cut down or eliminate sugars and highly refined cereals and processed foods. They clearly would have no problems with my advice to cut down on fatty meats and the types of fat (trans fats) found in margarines and many processed foods. They would be overjoyed about my recommendations to boost fresh fruit and vegetable consumption. But I can assure you that they would respond ferociously to the sheer thought of eliminating "hallowed" whole grains from your diet. If they heard I also advocate reducing or eliminating dairy products from your diet, they almost certainly would label this diet unhealthful, if not utterly dangerous. You may ask yourself, "Aren't whole grains healthful, and isn't milk good for everybody? How in the world can I get my calcium if I no longer eat dairy foods, and how can I get my fiber, B vitamins and other nutrients provided by whole grains?"

Whole Grains and Dairy Products: Nutritional Lightweights

One of the primary goals of any diet should be to supply you with a diet rich in nutrients (vitamins, minerals and phytochemicals) that promotes good health. Table 7.1 shows the nutrient density of seven

Table 7.1. Nutrient Density for Various Foods Groups (100 Kcal Samples).
Food Group Superscripts Represent Relative Ranking
(7 = Highest, 1 = Lowest) for Each Nutrient.

	Whole Grains	Whole Milk	Fruits	Veg.	Sea Food	Lean Meats	Nuts/ Seeds
Vitamin B12 (µg)	0.00^4	0.58^5	0.00^4	0.00^4	7.42^7	0.63^6	0.00^4
Vitamin B3 (mg)	1.12^4	0.14^1	0.89^3	2.73^5	3.19^6	4.73^7	0.35^2
Phosphorus (mg)	90^3	152^5	33^1	157^6	219^7	151^4	80^2
Vitamin B2 (mg)	0.05^2	0.26^6	0.09^3	0.33^7	0.09^4	0.14^5	0.04^1
Vitamin B1 (mg)	0.12^5	0.06^1	0.11^3	0.26^7	0.08^2	0.18^6	0.12^4
Folate (µg)	10.3^4	8.1^2	25.0^6	208.3^7	10.8^3	3.8^1	11.0^5
Vitamin C (mg)	0.0^1	74.2^4	221.3^6	93.6^7	1.9^5	0.1^2	0.4^3
Iron (mg)	0.90^4	0.08^1	0.69^2	2.59^7	2.07^6	1.10^5	0.86^3
Vitamin B6 (mg)	0.09^3	0.07^1	0.20^5	0.42^7	0.19^4	0.32^6	0.08^2
Vitamin A (RE)	2^2	50^5	94^6	687^7	32^4	1^1	2^3
Magnesium (mg)	32.6^4	21.9^2	24.6^3	54.5^7	36.1^6	18.0^1	35.8^5
Calcium (mg)	7.6^2	194.3^7	43.0^4	116.8^6	43.1^5	6.1^1	17.5^3
Zinc (mg)	0.67^4	0.62^3	0.25^1	1.04^5	7.6^7	1.9^6	0.6^2
Sum Rank Score	**42**	**43**	**47**	**82**	**66**	**51**	**39**

*Nutrient values represent average of food types within each food group: 8 whole grains, 20 fruits, 18 vegetables, 20 types of seafood, 4 lean meats, 10 seeds and nuts. Food types within food groups were based upon the most commonly consumed foods in the U.S. diet for the 13 vitamins and minerals most frequently lacking or deficient in the U.S. diet.

foods groups. From top to bottom, here's the ranking of the most nutritious food groups: #1 fresh vegetables, #2 seafood, #3 lean meats, # 4 fresh fruits, #5 whole milk, #6 whole grains, #7 nuts and seeds. It should now be obvious to you that whole grains and dairy foods are not nearly as nutritious as they are frequently stacked up to be. In fact, these foods are nutritional lightweights. Your diet will not suffer in the least by avoiding dairy and cereals. In reality, the exact opposite will be true. You will be getting more vitamins, minerals and phytochemicals when you increase your consumption of fresh fruit, veggies, lean meats, fish and seafood.

Whole Grains and Fiber

How about fiber? I'm sure that you've heard that whole grains are great sources of fiber. Right? Wrong again! Take a look at Figure 7.1 below and you can see that whole grains can't hold a candle to the fiber content of fruits and vegetables. Moreover, fresh fruits and veggies contain primarily soluble fiber that can help to lower your blood cholesterol levels, whereas except for oats, whole grains are poor sources

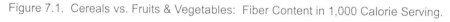

Figure 7.1. Cereals vs. Fruits & Vegetables: Fiber Content in 1,000 Calorie Serving.

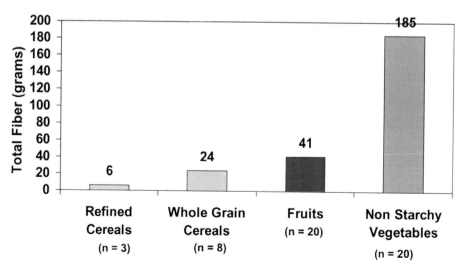

of soluble fiber. When you replace whole grains with fresh fruits and veggies, the fiber content of your diet will not suffer, but rather will increase.

Calcium and Milk

One of your biggest concerns when you avoid or eliminate dairy products may be this question, "How am I going to get my calcium?" Now if you have been swayed by those milk mustache ads, you probably are part of the mass hysteria, largely generated by the dairy industry, suggesting there is a nation-wide calcium shortage that underlies osteoporosis. Not true! Calcium intake from dairy, or any other food, is only part of the story behind bone mineral health. More important is calcium balance, the difference between how much calcium you've got coming into your body from diet, and the amount leaving in the urine. You will be out of calcium balance if more calcium leaves your body than what comes in, no matter how much milk you drink. What we really need to pay attention to is the other side of the calcium balance equation – the calcium leaving our bodies.

Dietary acid/base balance is the single most important factor influencing calcium loss in the urine. Net acid producing diets overloaded with grains, cheeses and salty, processed foods increase urinary calcium losses, whereas the new diet you will be eating is rich in alkaline yielding fruits and vegetables that bring us back into calcium balance and promote bone mineral health.

Nutritional Superiority of "The Dietary Cure for Acne"

You now know that the diet you will be embarking upon contains no grains, no dairy products, no processed foods, and no fatty meats and consists almost entirely of fresh fruits, veggies, lean meats and seafood. The following table outlines a typical day for a 25-year-old woman consuming 2,200 calories.

Table 7.2. Sample 1-Day Menu from "The Dietary Cure for Acne" Diet for a 25 Year Old Female with a 2200 Kcal Daily Energy Intake.

BREAKFAST	Food Quantity (g)	Energy (kcal)
Cantaloupe	276	97
Atlantic salmon (broiled)	333	605
LUNCH		
Vegetable salad with walnuts		
Shredded Romaine lettuce	68	10
Sliced carrot	61	26
Sliced cucumber	78	10
Quartered tomatoes	246	52
Lemon juice dressing	31	8
Walnuts	11	70
Broiled lean pork loin	86	205
DINNER		
Vegetable avocado/almond salad		
Shredded mixed greens	112	16
Tomato	123	26
Avocado	85	150
Slivered almonds	45	260
Sliced red onion	29	11
Lemon juice dressing	31	8
Steamed broccoli	468	131
Lean beef sirloin tip roast	235	400
Dessert – Strawberries	130	39
SNACKS		
Orange	66	30
Carrot sticks	81	35
Celery sticks	90	14

Now let's see how this representative day's worth of modern Paleo food stacks up to the USDA Food Pyramid. First, let's take a look at the major dietary components which are listed in the Table 7.3 below.

Table 7.3. Comparison of the "Dietary Cure for Acne" Diet with the USDA Food Pyramid Diet for Females (25 Yrs, 2,200 Kcal Daily Energy Intake).

	Food Pyramid	Dietary Cure for Acne
Protein (g)	113	217
Protein (% energy)	20	38
Carbohydrate (g)	302	129
Carbohydrate (% energy)	53	23
Total sugars (g)	96.6	76.5
Fiber (g)	30.0	42.5
Fat (g)	67.0	100.3
Fat (% total energy)	27.0	39.0
Saturated fat (g)	19.6	18.0
Saturated fat (% total energy)	7.0	6.4
Monounsaturated fat (g)	22.8	44.3
Polyunsaturated fat (g)	19.0	26.7
Omega-3 fat (g)	1.0	9.6
Omega-6 fat (g)	14.3	14.2
Cholesterol (mg)	219	461
Sodium (mg)	2626	726
Potassium (mg)	3450	9062

You immediately see that "The Dietary Cure for Acne" is much higher in protein and lower in carbohydrate than the Food Pyramid diet. Even though more than half of the calories in our diet come from meat and seafood, the saturated fat content is quite low – even lower than recommended values (10%) known to reduce the risk for high blood cholesterol and heart disease. The fats you will be getting in this diet are just plain good for you! Notice the good fats (mono-unsaturated and polyunsaturated fats) which lower blood cholesterol levels are considerably higher than what you would get by following the Food Pyramid diet.

Omega-3 Fats

Most people have heard that omega-3 fats found in fish, like salmon, are healthful, but few are aware that a family of fats called omega-6 fats found in vegetable oils, margarine and processed foods can be harmful when consumed at the expense of omega-3 fats. In the standard American diet the ratio of omega-6 to omega-3 fats is an unhealthy 10 to 1. In contrast this ratio is a wholesome 2 to 1 in "The Dietary Cure for Acne". Now take a look at the Food Pyramid – their recommendation is an appalling (14 to 1) and is actually worse than what the average American is currently eating! The Food Pyramid was originally conceived and thrust upon a trusting U.S. public in 1992, prior to the widespread knowledge that an imbalance in omega-6 and 3 fats had so much to do with health and well-being. Unfortunately we are still saddled with this botched bit of advice – even in the most recent version of the Food Pyramid.

The average U.S. diet is deficient in omega-3 fatty acids and amounts to a paltry 1.6 grams per day of which 1.4 grams come from alpha linolenic acid (ALA), and only 0.1 to 0.2 grams come from EPA and DHA. Most of the beneficial effects of omega-3 fatty acids are due to EPA and DHA. Because the conversion of ALA to DHA and EPA in the liver is inefficient, very little ALA is converted to EPA and DHA. Try to include at least 0.5-1.8 grams of EPA + DHA per day in your diet. The foods that comprise 70% of the calories in the typical U.S. diet (refined sugars, cereal grains, dairy products, and refined vegetable oils) contain little or no EPA or DHA. The best dietary source of EPA and DHA is fish. In Table 7.4 below you can see which fish are highest in EPA and DHA.

Table 7.4. Omega-3 Fatty Acid Content in Fish and Seafood per 100 g Portion. ALA = alpha linolenic acid (18:3n3), EPA = eicosapentaenoic acid (20:5n3), DHA = docosahexaenoic acid (22:6n3), Tr = Trace amount.

FINFISH	ALA (g)	EPA (g)	DHA (g)	Total
Anchovy, European		0.5	0.9	1.4
Bass, freshwater	Tr	0.1	0.2	0.3
Bass, striped	Tr	0.2	0.6	0.8
Bluefish		0.4	0.8	1.2
Burbot	--	0.1	0.1	0.2
Carp	0.3	0.2	0.1	0.6
Catfish, brown bullhead	0.1	0.2	0.2	0.5
Catfish, channel	Tr	0.1	0.2	0.3
Cisco	0.1	0.1	0.3	0.5
Cod, Atlantic	Tr	0.1	0.2	0.3
Cod, Pacific	Tr	0.1	0.1	0.2
Croaker, Atlantic	Tr	0.1	0.1	0.2
Dogfish, spiny	0.1	0.7	1.2	2.0
Dolphin fish	Tr	Tr	0.1	0.1
Drum, black	Tr	0.1	0.1	0.2
Drum, freshwater	0.1	0.2	0.3	0.6
Eel, European	0.7	0.1	0.1	0.9
Flounder, unspecified	Tr	0.1	0.1	0.2
Flounder, yellowtail	Tr	0.1	0.1	0.2
Grouper, jewfish	Tr	Tr	0.3	0.3
Grouper, red	--	Tr	0.2	0.2

FINFISH	ALA (g)	EPA (g)	DHA (g)	Total
Haddock	Tr	0.1	0.1	0.2
Hake, Atlantic	Tr	Tr	Tr	0.0
Hake, Pacific	Tr	0.2	0.2	0.4
Hake, red	--	0.1	0.1	0.2
Hake, silver	0.1	0.2	0.3	0.6
Hake, unspecified	--	0.1	0.4	0.5
Halibut, Greenland	Tr	0.5	0.4	0.9
Halibut, Pacific	0.1	0.1	0.3	0.5
Herring, Atlantic	0.1	0.7	0.9	1.7
Herring, Pacific	0.1	1.0	0.7	1.8
Herring, round	0.1	0.4	0.8	1.3
Mackerel, Atlantic	0.1	0.9	1.6	2.6
Mackerel, chub	0.3	0.9	1.0	2.2
Mackerel, horse	Tr	0.3	0.3	0.6
Mackerel, Japanese horse	0.1	0.5	1.3	1.9
Mackerel, king	--	1.0	1.2	2.2
Mullet, striped	0.1	0.3	0.2	0.6
Mullet, unspecified	Tr	0.5	0.6	1.1
Ocean perch	Tr	0.1	0.1	0.2
Perch, white	0.1	0.2	0.1	0.4
Perch, yellow	Tr	0.1	0.2	0.3
Pike, northern	Tr	Tr	0.1	0.1
Pike, walleye	Tr	0.1	0.2	0.3
Plaice, European	Tr	0.1	0.1	0.2
Pollock	--	0.1	0.4	0.5
Pompano, Florida	--	0.2	0.4	0.6
Ratfish	Tr	Tr	0.1	0.1
Rockfish, brown	Tr	0.3	0.4	0.7
Rockfish, unspecified	Tr	0.2	0.3	0.5
Sablefish	0.1	0.7	0.7	1.5
Salmon, Atlantic	0.2	0.3	0.9	1.4

FINFISH	ALA (g)	EPA (g)	DHA (g)	Total
Salmon, Chinook	0.1	0.8	0.6	1.5
Salmon, Coho	0.2	0.3	0.5	1.0
Salmon, pink	Tr	0.4	0.6	1.0
Salmon, sockeye	0.1	0.5	0.7	1.3
Saury	0.1	0.5	0.8	1.4
Scad, Muroaji	0.1	0.5	1.5	2.1
Scad, other	--	Tr	Tr	0.0
Sea bass, Japanese	Tr	0.1	0.3	0.4
Sea trout, sand	Tr	0.1	0.2	0.3
Sea trout, spotted	Tr	0.1	0.1	0.2
Shark, unspecified	--	Tr	0.5	0.5
Sheepshead	Tr	0.1	0.1	0.2
Smelt, pond	--	0.1	0.2	0.3
Smelt, rainbow	0.1	0.3	0.4	0.8
Smelt, sweet	0.3	0.2	0.1	0.6
Snapper, red	Tr	Tr	0.2	0.2
Sole, European	Tr	Tr	0.1	0.1
Sprat	--	0.5	0.8	1.3
Sturgeon, Atlantic	Tr	1.0	0.5	1.5
Sturgeon, common	0.1	0.2	0.1	0.4
Sunfish, pumpkinseed	Tr	Tr	0.1	0.1
Swordfish	--	0.1	0.1	0.2
Trout, arctic char	Tr	0.1	0.5	0.6
Trout, brook	0.2	0.2	0.2	0.6
Trout, lake	0.4	0.5	1.1	2.0
Trout, rainbow	0.1	0.1	0.4	0.6
Tuna, albacore	0.2	0.3	1.0	1.5
Tuna, blue fin	--	0.4	1.2	1.6
Tuna, skipjack	0.1	0.3	0.4	
Tuna, unspecified	--	0.1	0.4	0.5
Whitefish, lake	0.2	0.3	1.0	1.5

Whiting, European	Tr	Tr	0.1		0.1
Wolfish, Atlantic	Tr	0.3	0.3		0.6

CRUSTACEANS

Crab, Alaska king	Tr	0.2	0.1		0.3
Crab, blue	T r	0.2	0.2		0.4
Crab, Dungeness	--	0.2	0.1		0.3
Crab, queen	Tr	0.2	0.1		0.3
Crayfish, unspecified	Tr	0.1	Tr		0.1
Lobster, European	0.1	0.1	0.2		
Lobster, northern	0.1	0.1	0.2		
Shrimp, Atlantic brown	Tr	0.2	0.1		0.3
Shrimp, Atlantic white	Tr	0.2	0.2		0.4
Shrimp, Japanese	Tr	0.3	0.2		0.5
Shrimp, northern	Tr	0.3	0.2		0.5
Shrimp, unspecified	Tr	0.2	0.1		0.3
Spiny lobster, Caribbean	Tr	0.2	0.1		0.3
Spiny lobster, S. Rock	Tr	0.2	0.1		0.3

MOLLUSKS

Abalone, South African	Tr	Tr	Tr		0.0
Clam, hard-shell	Tr	Tr	Tr		0.0
Clam, littleneck	Tr	Tr	Tr		0.0
Clam, Japanese hard-shell	--	0.1	0.1		0.2
Clam, soft-shell	Tr	0.2	0.2		0.4
Clam, surf	Tr	0.1	0.1		0.2
Conch, unspecified	Tr	0.6	0.4		1.0
Cuttlefish, unspecified	Tr	Tr	Tr		0.0
Mussel, blue	Tr	0.2	0.3		0.5
Mussel, Mediterranean	--	0.1	0.1		0.2
Octopus, common	--	0.1	0.1	0.1	0.2
Oyster, eastern	Tr	0.2	0.2	0.2	0.4

Oyster, European	0.1	0.3	0.2	0.6
Oyster, Pacific	Tr	0.4	0.2	0.6
Periwinkle, common	0.2	0.5	Tr	0.7
Scallop, Atlantic deep sea	Tr	0.1	0.1	0.2
Scallop, unspecified	Tr	0.1	0.1	0.2
Squid, Atlantic	Tr	0.1	0.3	0.4
Squid, short-finned	Tr	0.2	0.4	0.6
Squid, unspecified	Tr	0.1	0.2	0.3
FISH OILS				
Cod liver oil	0.7	9.0	9.5	19.2
Herring oil	0.6	7.1	4.3	12.0
Menhaden oil	1.1	12.7	7.9	21.7
Max EPA, concentrated	0	17.8	11.6	29.4

Glycemic Index and Glycemic Load

There are additional troubles with the Pyramid beyond its improper fat balance. In 1992, the concept of a glycemic load and how it impacts health was completely unknown to the dietitians who designed the Pyramid. Should we be concerned about the glycemic load of a food? Absolutely! Does the Food Pyramid differentiate high and low glycemic foods? Absolutely not – not even in the newly re-designed My Pyramid!

Vitamins and Minerals

Let's contrast the nutrient density of our example diet to the USDA Food Pyramid. Take a quick look at Table 7.5 on the next page and you will see that there is really no comparison. Except for calcium "The Dietary Cure for Acne" simply blows away the Food Pyramid. As I explained earlier in this chapter, a reduced calcium intake does not represent a problem, particularly if you eat ample fruits and vegetables.

Table 7.5. Trace Nutrients in "The Dietary Cure for Acne" Diet and in the USDA Food Pyramid Diet for Females (25 Yrs, 2,200 Kcal Daily Energy Intake).

	Food Pyramid		Acne Cure Diet	
		% DRI		% DRI
Vitamin A (RE)	1,659	207	6386	798
Vitamin B1 (mg)	2.3	209	3.4	309
Vitamin B2 (mg)	2.6	236	4.2	355
Vitamin B3 (mg)	30	214	60	428
Vitamin B6 (mg)	2.6	200	6.7	515
Folate (µg)	453	113	891	223
Vitamin B12 (µg)	4.7	196	17.6	733
Vitamin C (mg)	233	388	748	1247
Vitamin E (IU)	10	125	19.5	244
Calcium (mg)	1215	122	691	69
Phosphorus (mg)	1808	258	2546	364
Magnesium (mg)	427	138	643	207
Iron (mg)	19	127	24.3	162
Zinc (mg)	14	116	27.4	228

FOODS TO EAT

There really are no exotic foods that you'll need to buy to correctly follow "The Dietary Cure for Acne". No matter if you live in a big city or in the country, the mainstays of the diet (lean meats, fish, fresh fruits and vegetables) are almost always on hand at your local grocery store or supermarket. In Chapter 6 I've given you a wide-ranging list of the foods you should limit or eliminate from your diet. In this chapter, I'll show you all the delectable health giving foods you have the indulgence to eat.

Acceptable Fresh Vegetables:

The following list certainly is not comprehensive and nearly all fresh vegetables, except potatoes, are entirely acceptable. As I previously pointed out, potatoes maintain high glycemic loads and should be eaten sparingly or avoided.

The list: asparagus, parsnip, radish, broccoli, lettuce, mushrooms, dandelion, mustard greens, watercress, purslane, onions, green onions, carrots, parsley, squash of all varieties, bell peppers, all peppers, artichoke, tomato, cauliflower, cabbage, brussel sprouts, celery, cucumber, tomatillos, collards, Swiss chard, endive, beet greens, beets, turnips, rutabaga, kohlrabi, kale, eggplant, pumpkin, turnip greens, spinach, seaweed, yams

Sweet potatoes and yams should be avoided during the first 30 day run-in for the diet. Later you may want to add these starchy tubers back into your menu and see if they are OK and don't cause flare ups. Also, remember that corn on the cob is actually a grain and is therefore not part of the 30 day run-in diet. Similarly, green beans and peas should be initially avoided and then later added back to your diet to determine if they cause flare-ups.

Acceptable Fresh Fruit:

As was the case with vegetables, any fresh fruit you can get your hands on is fair game. The only exceptions are dried fruits (raisins, dates, figs, etc), which like potatoes should be avoided since they also have quite high glycemic loads.

The list: apples, oranges, pears, peaches, plums, kiwi fruit, pomegranate, grapes, watermelon, cantaloupe, cassava melon, pineapple, guava, nectarine, apricot, strawberry, blackberries, blueberries, raspberries, avocado, carambola, cherimoya, cherry, fig, grapefruit, lemon, lime, lychee, mango, papaya, passion fruit, persimmon, tangerine, star fruit, gooseberries, boysenberries, rhubarb, cranberries, honeydew melon, and all other fruits

Acceptable Meats, Poultry and Eggs

Lean beef: flank steak trimmed of visible fat, top sirloin steak trimmed of visible fat, extra lean ground beef (drain fat from pan when possible), London broil trimmed of visible fat, chuck steak trimmed of visible fat, all lean cuts trimmed of visible fat, lean beef jerky

Lean pork: lean pork loin, lean pork chops, lean pork roasts, all lean cuts trimmed of visible fat

Lean chicken, turkey and game hens: skinless breasts

Eggs: Eggs are actually a high fat food and a single egg averages 62% fat by energy. I recommend that you limit egg consumption to six per week and buy omega-3 enriched eggs whenever possible.

Organ Meats: Except for marrow and brains, the organs of commercially produced animals are quite lean. However, the liver and kidneys are organs that cleanse and de-toxify the animal's body and frequently may contain high concentrations of environmental contaminants. I recommend eating only calves liver because virtually all calves slaughtered in the U.S haven't found their way to the toxic feed lot environment, and hence all are pasture fed. Brains contain high concentrations of omega-3 fatty acids, but because of the small risk of developing Prion Disease (Mad Cow Disease), I do not advise eating the brains of any animal, domestic or wild. Cholesterol lowering monounsaturated fatty acids are the dominant (~65% of total fatty acids) fatty acids in marrow and tongue. Both of these organs are quite healthful and tasty. Beef, lamb and pork sweetbreads are also lean and contain healthful fatty acids.

Grass Fed or Free Ranging Meats: If you can find it grass fed, or free ranging, beef, pork and poultry will always be a better choice than domestic meat because it contains more of the healthful omega-3 fatty acids, is low in total fat, and is less likely to be contaminated with hormones and pesticides

Commercially Available Game Meat and Other Exotic Meats: In the U.S. the commercial sale of hunted, wild game is prohibited. So unless you are a hunter, the only way to obtain game meat is to purchase meat that has been produced on game farms or ranches. Generally, meat from these animals is superior to feed lot produced animals, but may not necessarily be as lean or healthful as completely wild game. It is not an uncommon practice to feed grain to elk and buffalo to fatten them before slaughter.

The list: kangaroo, venison, elk, alligator, reindeer, pheasant, quail, muscovy duck, goose, wild boar, ostrich, rattlesnake, emu, turtle, African Springbok antelope, New Zealand Cervena deer, squab, wild turkey, caribou, bear, buffalo, rabbit, goat

Acceptable Fish:

Fish can frequently contain high concentrations of mercury and pesticides. To minimize your risk of eating contaminated fish, avoid eating freshwater fish from lakes and rivers, particularly the Great Lakes and other industrialized areas. Also avoid large long-lived fish such as swordfish, tuna and shark as they tend to concentrate mercury in their flesh. If you cannot easily obtain fresh fish, water packed canned salmon, tuna and sardines are good second choices.

The list: salmon, halibut, herring, trout, catfish, bass, mackerel, cod, scrod, northern pike, sunfish, haddock, grouper, walleye, flatfish, red snapper, monkfish, rockfish, perch tilapia, striped bass, turbot, mullet, bluefish, drum, eel, orange roughy, or any other commercially available or fresh caught fish

Acceptable Shellfish:

The list: abalone, clams, crab, crayfish, lobster, mussels, oysters, scallops, shrimp, whelk or any other commercially available or fresh caught crustacean or mollusk

Acceptable Oils:

In Chapter 5 (Tables 5.2 and 5.3), I have already provided you with all the information you will need to pick out the best oils. Oils that you will use for cooking need to be stable and resistant to the oxidizing effects of heat, whereas the oils you use in your salads don't. Saturated fatty acids (SAT) are the most stable and heat resistant followed by monounsaturated fatty acids (MUFA), and then polyunsaturated fatty acids (PUFA). Because SAT elevate blood cholesterol levels, your choice of cooking oils should be high in MUFA and relatively low in both SAT and PUFA. Good choices for cooking include olive oil, avocado oil and canola oil. All oils, regardless of their fatty acid makeup, oxidize during cooking. Consequently, you should not fry at high or searing heats but rather, keep sautéing temperatures low to medium and cook for shorter periods.

The stability of any oil is determined not only by its relative ratio of SAT /MUFA /PUFA, but also by the type of PUFA. Omega-3 PUFA are more fragile than omega-6 PUFA. Consequently, flaxseed and walnut oil should not be used to cook with because of their high concentration of total PUFA and omega-3 PUFA. However, both of these oils are good choices for your salads. Flaxseed oil is the richest vegetable source of omega-3 fatty acids. It can be poured over steamed veggies or incorporated into a marinade that is added to meat and seafood after cooking. Both strategies are great ways to get more omega-3 fatty acids into your diet.

The only oils I recommend are flaxseed, canola, walnut, avocado and olive. Although soybean oil and wheat germ oils appear to have acceptable fatty acid balances, both are concentrated sources of lectins. Wheat germ oil is the highest dietary source of the lectin, wheat germ agglutinin (WGA) and soybean oil contains soybean agglutinin (SBA). Similarly, peanuts are really not nuts but rather legumes. Peanut oil, just like soybean oil, is a concentrated source of the lectin, peanut agglutinin (PNA). Because all of these dietary lectins can enter your bloodstream and adversely influence a number of the cellular and hormonal processes underlying the development of acne, I recommend that you strongly avoid these oils or any processed food products made with them.

Acceptable Nuts and Seeds:

As an acne patient, you will need to be cautious when it comes to nuts and seeds. As I have mentioned many times in this book, peanuts are not nuts but rather are legumes containing the lectin, PNA. Hence peanuts, peanut butter and peanut oil definitely need to be avoided during the 30 day run-in portion of the diet. If you absolutely are in love with peanuts or peanut butter, you may want to experiment with this food by adding it back into your diet in the months following the initial 30 day run-in.

Except for peanuts, nuts and seeds have been poorly studied when it comes to whether or not they contain lectins that can get past the gut and into the bloodstream. It is known that walnuts, hazelnuts and coconuts contain lectins that cause red blood cells in glass dishes to clump (agglutinate). However, no follow-up studies have ever been conducted to determine which specific lectins are involved or if they can enter the bloodstream. Many people have food allergies, and nuts are one of the more common ones. Always listen to your body, if you know or suspect that nuts do not agree with you – then don't eat them.

This advice holds for all foods, including shellfish, which also frequent-ly cause allergies.

In Table 5.3 you can see the fatty acid balance for most of the com-monly available nuts. Notice that except for walnuts, all other nuts maintain high omega-6 to omega-3 ratios. The ideal omega-6/ omega-3 ratio in your diet should be about 2:1 or slightly lower. Because nuts are so calorically dense they can very easily de-rail the best laid dietary plans and give you too much omega-6 fatty acids. You recall from Chapter 5 that excessive omega-6 fatty acids can cause inflammation which is a key component underlying acne. Enjoy nuts, but use them sparingly.

SUPPLEMENTS

FISH OIL CAPSULES

Some people just don't like fish, and there is no way they could ever get the recommended intake of omega-3 fats from eating fish. If you are like these people, I suggest that you supplement your diet with fish oil capsules. During the first 30 day period of the diet, I recommend that you take between 2-4 grams of both EPA and DHA daily. This amount of fish oil will help to rapidly calm your overly agitated inflam-matory response and get your skin on the road to recovery. After the 30 day run-in, try to include at least 0.5-1.8 grams of EPA + DHA per day in your diet, either by eating fish or by taking fish oil supplements.

ZINC

In addition to fish oil capsules, I recommend that you supplement your daily diet with 50 mg of zinc gluconate. Many acne patients have consumed diets for years and years that do not meet the daily recom-mended intake (12 to15 mg) of zinc. Hence, supplementation of this vital mineral will help to calm inflammation and may also facilitate the normal desquamation (shedding) of corneocytes so that they will not block the opening (pore) of the follicle.

Quite often, in the U.S., we think that if a little bit of something is good, then a whole lot must be better. Definitely not the case for zinc! Excess zinc supplementation (>100 mg per day) for extended periods frequently results in a copper deficiency. Consequently, for the first 30 days of the program, I recommend that you supplement your normal daily diet with 50 mg of zinc, and then back down to 25 mg after the initial run-in. With your new diet you will be eating lots of zinc rich foods (lean red meats), while simultaneously avoiding zinc- poor foods (refined sugars, refined grains, and vegetable oils) and foods that impair zinc absorption (legumes, whole grains and dairy products). Consequently, zinc deficiency and its adverse effects upon your acne symptoms will become a thing of the past.

Vitamin D

The final dietary supplement I suggest that you take is vitamin D. This vitamin is really not a vitamin at all, but rather is a hormone that is normally produced in your skin when ultraviolet radiation from sunlight strikes cholesterol within the skin. Except for fish liver oil, almost all naturally occurring foods contain miniscule or no vitamin D. Starting in the 1950s, in the U.S. and elsewhere, food manufacturers began to fortify milk and margarine with vitamin D. Accordingly, before milk and margarine were fortified with vitamin D, almost every human on the planet was dependent upon sunshine to obtain this vital substance. Because I do not recommend that you drink milk or eat margarine with "The Dietary Cure for Acne", you will need to supplement your daily diet with 1,000 I.U. of vitamin D. The only exception to this general rule of thumb would be if you are currently living in a warm climate where you can get daily sunshine exposure.

RECIPES

When you have the choice, always choose your foods in this order: 1) fresh foods, 2) frozen foods, 3) canned foods. When you prepare recipes from common every day foods you can get in the supermarket, keep in mind you want to make sure the ingredients are free of: 1) grains 2) dairy products, 3) refined sugars 4) legumes, including peanuts, 5) yeast and yeast containing foods such as baked goods, pickled foods, vinegar, fermented foods and fermented beverages and 6) contain only permitted oils. Remember to select the leanest cuts of meats and trim away any visible fat. Keep in mind, the foundation of this diet is lean meats, seafood, fresh fruits and veggies.

If you visit my website: www.ThePaleoDiet.com, and click on the nutrition icon and then on the recipes icon www.ThePaleoDiet.com/nutritional_tools/recipes.shtml you will now have more than 100 delicious recipes to help you get started eating in this new way. I have included recipes for: 1) Seafood, 2) Domestic Low-Fat Meat Entrees (Beef, Pork, Chicken), 3) Organ Meat Entrees, 4) Game Meat Entrees, 6) Dried Meats (Jerky), 7) Vegetable Dishes, 8) Salads, 9) Condiments, Dips, Salsas, Salad Dressings, Marinades, 10) Soups, and 11) Fruit Dishes and Desserts.

So, start your way to a new you. In 30 days, you can dramatically improve or eliminate your acne. The new foods that you will be adding to your diet will not only improve your acne, but these foods will give you added energy and will enhance your overall health and well being. The "Dietary Cure for Acne" is not a diet at all, but rather a healthful, lifelong way of eating. Enjoy!

THE BOTTOM LINE

- By eliminating whole grains and dairy foods from your diet and replacing them with fresh fruits, vegetables, lean meats, fish and seafood, you will actually increase the vitamins, minerals and fiber in your diet.

- By increasing your intake of fresh fruits and vegetables and by avoiding or eliminating processed foods made with refined sugars, grains and vegetable oils, your diet will be net alkaline yielding, thereby promoting calcium balance and good bone mineral health, despite the lack of dairy foods in your diet.

- To promote more rapid clearing of your acne symptoms I suggest that you supplement your diet with fish oil capsules (2-4 grams of DHA + EPA) and zinc (50 mg) for the initial 30 day run-in.

- Margarine and milk are fortified with vitamin D because there is little or no vitamin D in everyday foods. We naturally make vitamin D in our skins, following sunlight exposure. However, if you don't get regular sun, I recommend that you take 1,000 I.U. of vitamin D daily.

- There are no exotic foods required for this diet to work. All of the foods that you will need to improve your acne such as fresh fruits, vegetables, lean meats, fish and seafood are easily obtainable at your local supermarket.

More than 100 delicious recipes, snacks and ideas for your new way of eating are available at:

www.ThePaleoDiet.com/nutritional_tools/recipes.shtml

Reader Feedback

The advent of the internet and electronic down-loadable e-books has now opened up brand new avenues for the book writing process and made interaction between readers and author much easier. After trying "The Dietary Cure for Acne" for 30 days, feel free to send us your comments at: feedback@DietaryAcneCure.com . Though I cannot personally reply to all emails, I encourage readers to share with me their questions and stories. In turn, I will answer some of the more interesting questions and share the successes of other readers in our newsletter and our website: www.DietaryAcneCure.com .

A preview of the book is available at our website as a free download to all interested persons. It's time to get the word out. Diet indeed causes acne!

SCIENTIFIC REFERENCES

1. Thiboutot DM, Strauss JS: Diseases of the sebaceous glands, in Freedberg IM, EisenAZ, Wolff K et al (Eds): Fitzpatrick's Dermatology in General Medicine, vol 1 (Ed 6). New York, NY, McGraw-Hill, 2003, p 683.

2. Cunliffe WJ, Simpson NB: Disorders of sebaceous glands, in Champion RH, S. Wilkinson DS, F. J. G. Ebling FJG et al (Eds): Rook/Wilkinson/Ebling Textbook of Dermatology, (ed 6). Oxford, Blackwell Science, Ltd, 1998, p. 1951.

3. Green J, Sinclair RD: Perceptions of acne vulgaris in final year medical student written examination answers. Austral J Dermatol 42:98-101, 2001

4. Loeffel ED: Foods and acne. J Tenn Med Assoc 65:918, 1972

5. Kaminester LH: Acne. JAMA 239:2171-2, 1978

6. Michaelsson G: Diet and acne. Nutr Rev 39:104-06, 1981

7. Rasmussen JE: Diet and acne. Int J Dermatol 16: 488-92, 1977

8. Bershad S: The unwelcome return of the acne diet. Arch Dermatol 139: 940-1, 2003

9. Smolinski KN, Yan AC: Acne update: 2004. Curr Opin Pediatr 16:385-91, 2004

10. Lehmann HP, Robinson KA, Andrews JS, et al: Acne therapy: a methodologic review. J Am Acad Dermatol 47:231-40, 2002

11. Anderson PC: Foods as the cause of acne. Am J Fam Pract 3: 102-3, 1971

12. Fulton JE, Plewig G, Kligman AM: Effect of chocolate on acne vulgaris. JAMA 210:2071-4, 1969

13. Treloar V: Diet and acne redux. Arch Dermatol 139:941, 2003

14. Cordain L: In reply. Arch Dermatol 139:942-3, 2003

15. Burkhart CN, Gottwald L: Assessment of etiologic agents in acne pathogenesis. Skinmed 2:222-28, 2003

16. Mullins JF, Naylor D: Glucose and the acne diathesis: an hypothesis

and review of pertinent literature. Tex Rep Biol Med 20:161-75, 1962

17. Foster-Powell K, Holt SH, Brand-Miller JC: International table of glycemic index and glycemic load values: 2002. Am J Clin Nutr 76:5-56, 2002

18. Gollnick H: Current concepts of the pathogenesis of acne. Drugs 63:1579-96, 2003

19. Cunliffe WJ, Holland DB, Clark SM, et al: Comedogenesis: some aetiological, clinical and therapeutic strategies. Dermatology206:11-16, 2003

20. Harper JC, Thiboutot DM: Pathogenesis of acne: recent research advances. Adv Dermatol19:1-10, 2003

21. Pawin H, Beylot C, Chivot M, et al: Physiopathology of acne vulgaris: recent data, new understanding of the treatments. Eur J Dermatol 14:4-12, 2004

22. Pochi PE, Shalita AR, Strauss JS et al: Report of the Consensus Conference on Acne Classification. Washington, D.C., March 24 and 25, 1990. J Am Acad Dermatol 24:495-500, 1991

23. White GM: Recent findings in the epidemiologic evidence, classification, and subtypes of acne vulgaris. J Am Acad Dermatol 39(2 Pt 3): S34-S37, 1998

24. Goulden V, Stables GI, Cunliffe WJ: Prevalence of facial acne in adults. J Am Acad Dermatol 41:577-580, 1999

25. Rademaker M, Garioch JJ, Simpson NB: Acne in schoolchildren: no longer a concern for dermatologists. Brit Med J 298:1217-1219, 1989

26. Kilkenny M, Merlin K, Plunkett A, et al: The prevalence of common skin conditions in Australian school students: 3. acne vulgaris. Br J Dermatol 139:840-845, 1998

27. Lello J, Pearl A, Arroll B, et al: Prevalence of acne vulgaris in Auckland senior high school students. N Z Med J 108:287-289, 1995

28. Hansman FS: Biochemistry in relation to the aetiology of acne vulgaris. Aust J Dermatol 1:120-24, 1951

29. Schaefer O: When the Eskimo comes to town. Nutr Today 6 (Nov/Dec):8-16, 1971

30. Steiner PE: Necropsies on Okinawans. Anatomic and pathologic observations. Arch Pathol 42:359-380, 1946

31. Cordain L, Lindeberg S, Hurtado M, et al: Acne vulgaris: a disease of Western civilization. Arch Dermatol138:1584-90, 2002

32. Goulden V, McGeown CH, Cunliffe WJ: The familial risk of adult acne: a comparison between first-degree relatives of affected and unaffected individuals. Br J Dermatol 141:297-300, 1999

33. Toyoda M, Morohashi M: Pathogenesis of acne. Med Electron Microsc 34:29-40, 2001

34. Oh CW, Myung KB: An ultra structural study of the retention hyperkeratosis of experimentally induced comedones in rabbits: the effects of three comedolytics. J Dermatol 23:169-80, 1996

35. Maeda T: An electron microscopic study of experimentally-induced comedo and effects of vitamin A acid on comedo formation. J Dermatol 18:397-407, 1991

36. Zelickson AS, Strauss JS, Mottaz J: Ultra structural changes in open comedones following treatment of cystic acne with isotretinoin. Am J Dermatopathol 7:241-4,1985.

37. Woo-Sam PC: The effect of vitamin A acid on experimentally induced comedones: an electron microscope study. Br J Dermatol 100:267-76, 1979

38. Woo-Sam PC: Cohesion of horny cells during comedo formation. An electron microscope study. Br J Dermatol 97:609-15, 1977

39. Knaggs HE, Holland DB, Morris C, et al: Quantification of cellular proliferation in acne using the monoclonal antibody Ki-67. J Invest Dermatol 102:89-92, 1994

40. Jenkins DJ, Wolever TM, Taylor RH, et al: Glycemic index of foods: a physiological basis for carbohydrate exchange. Am J Clin Nutr 34:362-6, 1981

41. Liu S, Willett WC: Dietary glycemic load and atherothrombotic risk.

Curr Atheroscler Rep 4:454-61, 2002

42. Foster-Powell K, Holt SH, Brand-Miller JC: International table of glycemic index and glycemic load values: 2002. Am J Clin Nutr 76:5-56, 2002

43. Holt SH, Miller JC, Petocz P: An insulin index of foods: the insulin demand generated by 1000-kJ portions of common foods. Am J Clin Nutr 66:1264-76, 1997

44. Ostman EM, Liljeberg Elmstahl HG, Bjorck IM: Inconsistency between glycemic and insulinemic responses to regular and fermented milk products. Am J Clin Nutr 74:96-100, 2001

45. Gerrior S, Bente L: Nutrient Content of the U.S. Food Supply, 1909-99: A Summary Report. U.S. Department of Agriculture, Center for Nutrition Policy and Promotion. Home Economics Report No. 55, 2002

46. Kiens B, Richter EA: Types of carbohydrate in an ordinary diet affect insulin action and muscle substrates in humans. Am J Clin Nutr 63:47-53, 1996

47. Ludwig DS: The glycemic index: physiological mechanisms relating to obesity, diabetes, and cardiovascular disease. JAMA 8; 287:2414-23, 2002

48. Liu S, Willett WC: Dietary glycemic load and atherothrombotic risk. Curr Atheroscler Rep 4:454-61, 2002

49. Edmondson SR, Thumiger SP, Werther GA, et al: Epidermal homeostasis: the role of the growth hormone and insulin-like growth factor systems. Endocr Rev 24:737-64, 2003

50. Nam SY, Lee EJ, Kim KR, et al: Effect of obesity on total and free insulin-like growth factor (IGF)-1, and their relationship to IGF-binding protein (BP)-1, IGFBP-2, IGFBP-3, insulin, and growth hormone. Int J Obes Relat Metab Disord 21:355-359, 1997

51. Attia N, Tamborlane WV, Heptulla R, et al: The metabolic syndrome and insulin-like growth factor I regulation in adolescent obesity. J Clin Endocrinol Metab 83:1467-1471, 1998

52. Brismar K, Fernqvist-Forbes E, Wahren J, et al: Effect of insulin on the hepatic production of insulin-like growth factor-binding protein-1 (IGFBP-1), IGFBP-3, and IGF-1 in insulin dependent diabetes. J Clin Endocrinol Metab 79:872-878, 1994

53. Holly JMP: The physiological role of IGFBP-1. Acta Endocrinol 124:55-62, 1991

54. Wong WW, Copeland KC, Hergenroeder AC, et al: Serum concentrations of insulin, insulin-like growth factor-I and insulin-like growth factor binding proteins are different between white and African American girls. J Pediatr 135:296-300, 1999

55. Loche S, Cappa M, Borrelli P, et al: Reduced growth hormone response to growth hormone-releasing hormone in children with simple obesity: evidence for somatomedin-C mediated inhibition. Clin Endocrinol (Oxf) 27:145-53, 1987

56. Liu VR: The Glycemic index and the insulin-like growth factor system. Honours Thesis. Human Nutrition Unit, Department of Biochemistry, University of Sydney, Sydney, Australia, 2000

57. Boden G, Shulman GI: Free fatty acids in obesity and type 2 diabetes: defining their role in the development of insulin resistance and beta-cell dysfunction. Eur J Clin Invest 32 Suppl 3:14-23, 2002

58. Vacaresse N, Lajoie-Mazenc I, Auge N, et al: Activation of epithelial growth factor receptor pathway by unsaturated fatty acids. Circ Res 85:892-9, 1999

59. Wolever TM, Mehling C: Long-term effect of varying the source or amount of dietary carbohydrate on postprandial plasma glucose, insulin, triacylglycerol, and free fatty acid concentrations in subjects with impaired glucose tolerance. Am J Clin Nutr 77:612-21, 2003

60. Lee KW, Cohen P: Nuclear effects: unexpected intracellular actions of insulin-like growth factor binding protein-3. J Endocrinol 175:33-40, 2002

61. Barbieri RL, Smith S, Ryan KJ: The role of hyperinsulinemia in the pathogenesis of ovarian hyperandrogenism. Fertil Steril 50:197-212,

1998

62. Cara JF: Insulin-like growth factors, insulin-like growth factor binding proteins and ovarian androgen production. Horm Res 42:49-54, 1994

63. Bebakar WM, Honour JW, Foster D, et al: Regulation of testicular function by insulin and transforming growth factor-beta. Steroids 55:266-270, 1990

64. De Mellow JS, Handelsman DJ, Baxter RC: Short-term exposure to insulin-like growth factors stimulates testosterone production by testicular interstitial cells. Acta Endocrinol 115:483-489, 1987

65. Crave JC, Lejeune H, Brebant C, et al: Differential effects of insulin and insulin-like growth factor I on the production of plasma steroid-binding globulins by human hepatoblastoma-derived (Hep G2) cells. J Clin Endocrinol Metab 80:1283-1289, 1995

66. Singh A, Hamilton-Fairley D, Koistinen R, et al: Effect of insulin-like growth factor-type I (IGF-I) and insulin on the secretion of sex hormone binding globulin and IGF-I binding protein (IBP-I) by human hepatoma cells. J Endocrinol 124:R1-R3, 1990

67. Pugeat M, Crave JC, Elmidani M, et al: Pathophysiology of sex hormone binding globulin (SHBG): relation to insulin. J Steroid Biochem Mol Biol 40:841-849, 1991

68. Vermeulen A, Kaufman JM, Giagulli VA: Influence of some biological indexes on sex hormone-binding globulin and androgen levels in aging or obese males. J Clin Endocrinol Metab 81:1821-1826, 1996

69. Pfeilschifter J, Scheidt-Nave C, Leidig-Bruckner G, et al: Relationship between circulating insulin-like growth factor components and sex hormones in a population-based sample of 50- to 80-year-old men and women. J Clin Endocrinol Metab 81:2534-2540, 1996

70. Erfurth EM, Hagmar LE, Saaf M, et al: Serum levels of insulin-like growth factor I and insulin-like growth factor-binding protein 1 correlate with serum free testosterone and sex hormone binding globulin levels in healthy young and middle-aged men. Clin Endocrinol 44:659-

664, 1996

71. Zouboulis CC, Xia L, Akamatsu H, et al: The human sebocyte culture model provides new insights into development and management of seborrhoea and acne. Dermatology 196:21-31, 1998

72. Deplewski D, Rosenfield RL: Growth hormone and insulin-like growth factors have different effects on sebaceous cell growth and differentiation. Endocrinology 140:4089-94, 1999

73. Klinger B, Anin S, Silbergeld A, et al: Development of hyperandrogenism during treatment with insulin-like growth hormone factor-I (IGF-1) in female patients with Laron syndrome. Clin Endocrinol 48:81-87, 1998

74. Thiboutot D, Gilliland K, Light J, et al: Androgen metabolism in sebaceous glands from subjects with and without acne. Arch Dermatol 135:1041-1045, 1999

75. Aizawa H, Niimura M: Elevated serum insulin-like growth factor-I (IGF-1) levels in women with postadolescent acne. J Dermatol 22:249-252, 1995

76. Aizawa H, Niimura M: Mild insulin resistance during oral glucose tolerance test (OGTT) in women with acne. J Dermatol 23:526-529, 1996

77. Vowels BR, Yang S, Leyden JJ: Induction of proinflammatory cytokines by a soluble factor of Propionibacterium acnes: implications for chronic inflammatory acne. Infect Immun 63:3158-65, 1995

78. Webster GF, Leyden JJ, Tsai CC, et al: Polymorphonuclear leukocyte lysosomal release in response to Propionibacterium acnes in vitro and its enhancement by sera from inflammatory acne patients. J Invest Dermatol 74:398-401, 1980

79. Norris JF, Cunliffe WJ: A histological and immunocytochemical study of early acne lesions. Br J Dermatol 118:651-9, 1988

80. Guy R, Kealey T: Modeling the infundibulum in acne. Dermatology. 196:32-7, 1998

81. Simopoulos AP: Omega-3 fatty acids in inflammation and autoim-

mune diseases.
J Am Coll Nutr 21:495-505, 2002

82. Kris-Etherton PM, Taylor DS, Yu-Poth S, et al: Polyunsaturated fatty acids in the food chain in the United States. Am J Clin Nutr 71(1 Suppl):179S-88S, 2000

83. Cordain L, Watkins BA, Florant GL, et al: Fatty acid analysis of wild ruminant tissues: Evolutionary implications for reducing diet-related chronic disease. Eur J Clin Nutr 56:181-91, 2002

84. Endres S, Ghorbani R, Kelley VE, et al: The effect of dietary supplementation with n-3 polyunsaturated fatty acids on the synthesis of interleukin-1 and tumor necrosis factor by mononuclear cells. N Engl J Med 320:265-71, 1989

85. Meydani SN, Endres S, Woods MM, et al: Oral (n-3) fatty acid supplementation suppresses cytokine production and lymphocyte proliferation: comparison between young and older women. J Nutr 121:547-55, 1991

86. James MJ, Gibson RA, Cleland LG: Dietary polyunsaturated fatty acids and inflammatory mediator production. Am J Clin Nutr 71(1 Suppl):343S-8S, 2000

87. Trebble T, Arden NK, Stroud MA, et al: Inhibition of tumour necrosis factor-alpha and interleukin 6 production by mononuclear cells following dietary fish-oil supplementation in healthy men and response to antioxidant co-supplementation. Br J Nutr 90:405-12, 2003

88. Zhao Y, Joshi-Barve S, Barve S, et al: Eicosapentaenoic acid prevents LPS-induced TNF-alpha expression by preventing NF-kappaB activation. J Am Coll Nutr 23:71-8, 2004

89. Mayer K, Meyer S, Reinholz-Muhly M, et al: Short-time infusion of fish oil-based lipid emulsions, approved for parenteral nutrition, reduces monocyte proinflammatory cytokine generation and adhesive interaction with endothelium in humans. J Immuno. 171:4837-43, 2003

90. Zouboulis CC, Nestoris S, Adler YD et al: Treatment of inflammatory acne with an oral 5-lipoxygenase inhibitor. J Invest Dermatol

117:547, 2001

Cohen JL, Cohen AD: Pustular acne, staphyloderma and its treatment with tolbutamide. Can Med Assoc J 80:629-632, 1959

91. Bettley FR: The treatment of acne vulgaris with tolbutamide. Br J Dermatol 1961; 73:149-151.

92. Singh I, Gaind ML, Jayram D. Tolbutamide in the treatment of skin diseases. Br J Dermatol 73:362-366, 1961

93. Depaoli M, Martina G: The therapeutic action of tolbutamide in common acne and acne rosacea. Panimnerva Med 365-66, 1961

94. Flinn JH: The treatment of acne with tolbutamide. Stud Med 9:234-7, 1961

95. Rustenbeck I: Desensitization of insulin secretion. Biochem Pharmacol 63:1921-35, 2002

96. Falsetti L, Eleftheriou Gl: Hyperinsulinemia in the polycystic ovary syndrome: a clinical endocrine and echographic study in 240 patients. Gynecol Endocrinol 10:319-326, 1996

97. Nestler JE: Insulin regulation of human ovarian androgens. Hum Reprod 12 (suppl 1): 53-62, 1997

98. Thierry van Dessel HJ, Lee PD, Faessen G, et al: Elevated serum levels of free insulin like growth factor-I levels in polycystic ovary syndrome. J Clin Endocrinol Metab 84:3030-35, 1999

99. Pasquali R, Casimirri F, Vicennati V: Weight control and its beneficial effect on fertility in women with obesity and polycystic ovary syndrome. Hum Reprod 12 (Suppl 1):82-87, 1997

100. Ehrmann DA: Insulin-lowering therapeutic modalities for polycystic ovary syndrome. Endocrinol Metab Clin North Am 28:423-38, 1999

101. Kolodziejczyk B, Duleba AJ, Spaczynski RZ, et al: Metformin therapy decreases hyperandrogenism and hyperinsulinemia in women with polycystic ovary syndrome. Fertil Steril 73:1149-54, 2000

102. Romualdi D, Guido M, Ciampelli M, et al: Selective effects of pioglitazone on insulin and androgen abnormalities in normo- and hyperinsulinaemic obese patients with polycystic ovary syndrome. Hum

Reprod 18:1210-8, 2003

103. Arslanian SA, Lewy V, Danadian K, et al: Metformin therapy in obese adolescents with polycystic ovary syndrome and impaired glucose tolerance: amelioration of exaggerated adrenal response to adrenocorticotropin with reduction of insulinemia/insulin resistance. J Clin Endocrinol Metab 87:1555-9, 2002

104. Guido M, Romualdi D, Suriano R, et al: Effect of pioglitazone treatment on the adrenal androgen response to corticotrophin in obese patients with polycystic ovary syndrome. Hum Reprod 19:534-9, 2004

105. Bourne S, Jacobs A: Observations on acne, seborrhea, and obesity. Br Med J 1:1268-70, 1956

106. Berrino F, Bellati C, Secreto G, et al: Reducing bioavailable sex hormones through a comprehensive change in diet: the diet and androgens (DIANA) randomized trial. Cancer Epidemiol Biomarkers Prev 10:25-33, 2001.

107. Adebamowo CA, Spiegelman D, Danby FW, Frazier AL, Willett WC, Holmes MD. High school dietary dairy intake and teenage acne. J Am Acad Dermatol. 2005 Feb; 52(2):207-14

108. Smith R, Mann N, Makelainen H, Braue A, Varigos G. The effect of short-term altered macronutrient status on acne vulgaris and biochemical markers of insulin sensitivity. Asia Pac J Clin Nutr. 2004; 13(Suppl):S67.

109. Smith R, Mann N, Braue A, Varigos G. The effect of a low glycemic load, high protein diet on hormonal markers of acne. Asia Pac J Clin Nutr. 2005; 14 Suppl: S43

110. Smith R, Mann N, Braue A, Varigos G. Low glycemic load, high protein diet lessens facial acne severity. Asia Pac J Clin Nutr. 2005; 14 Suppl: S97.

111. Cordain L, Eades MR, Eades MD. Hyperinsulinemic diseases of civilization: more than just syndrome X. Comp Biochem Physiol Part A 2003; 136:95-112.

112. Cordain L, Eaton SB, Sebastian A, Mann N, Lindeberg S, Watkins

BA, O'Keefe JH, Brand-Miller J. Origins and evolution of the western diet: Health implications for the 21st century. Am J Clin Nutr 2005; 81:341-54.

113. Hoyt G, Hickey MS, Cordain L. Dissociation of the glycaemic and insulinaemic responses to whole and skimmed milk. Br J Nutr 2005; 93:175-177.

114. Cordain, L. Implications for the role of diet in acne. Semin Cutan Med Surg 2005;24:84-91.

115. Amiel SA, Sherwin RS, Simonson DC, Lauritano AA, Tamborlane WV. Impaired insulin action in puberty. A contributing factor to poor glycemic control in adolescents with diabetes. N Engl J Med. 1986 Jul 24; 315(4):215-9

116. Moran A, Jacobs DR Jr, Steinberger J, Hong CP, Prineas R, Luepker R, Sinaiko AR.
Insulin resistance during puberty: results from clamp studies in 357 children. Diabetes. 1999 Oct; 48(10):2039-44

117. Poulton EP (Ed.). Taylor's Practice of Medicine, J.A. Churchill Ltd, London, 1936, p.861.

118. Dreno B, Foulc P, Reynaud A, Moyse D, Habert H, Richet H. Effect of zinc gluconate on propionibacterium acnes resistance to erythromycin in patients with inflammatory acne: in vitro and in vivo study. Eur J Dermatol. 2005 May-Jun;15(3):152-5

119. Dreno B, Trossaert M, Boiteau HL, Litoux P. Zinc salts effects on granulocyte zinc concentration and chemotaxis in acne patients. Acta Derm Venereol. 1992 Aug; 72(4):250-2.

120. Meynadier J. Efficacy and safety study of two zinc gluconate regimens in the treatment of inflammatory acne. Eur J Dermatol. 2000 Jun; 10(4):269-73.

121. Castillo-Duran, Solomons NW. Studies on the bioavailability of zinc in humans. IX. Interaction of beef-zinc with iron, calcium and lactose. Nutr Res 1991;11:429-38.

122. Savagner P, Yamada KM, Thiery JP. The zinc-finger protein

slug causes desmosome dissociation, an initial and necessary step for growth factor-induced epithelial-mesenchymal transition. J Cell Biol. 1997 Jun 16;137(6):1403-19

123. Skerrow CJ, Clelland DG, Skerrow D. Changes to desmosomal antigens and lectin-binding sites during differentiation in normal human epidermis: a quantitative ultrastructural study. J Cell Sci. 1989 Apr; 92 (Pt 4):667-77.

124. Schaumburg-Lever G. Ultrastructural localization of lectin-binding sites in normal skin. J Invest Dermatol. 1990 Apr; 94(4):465-70

125. Burge SM, Schomberg KH. Adhesion molecules and related proteins in Darier's disease and Hailey-Hailey disease. Br J Dermatol. 1992 Oct; 127(4):335-43.

126. Simon M, Montezin M, Guerrin M, Durieux JJ, Serre G. Characterization and purification of human corneodesmosin, an epidermal basic glycoprotein associated with corneocyte-specific modified desmosomes J Biol Chem. 1997 Dec 12;272(50):31770-6.

127. Milstone LM. Epidermal desquamation. J Dermatol Sci. 2004 Dec;36(3):131-40

128. Wang Q, Yu LG, Campbell BJ, Milton JD, Rhodes JM. Identification of intact peanut lectin in peripheral venous blood. Lancet. 1998 Dec 5; 352(9143):1831-2.

129. Pusztai A, Greer F, Grant G. Specific uptake of dietary lectins into the systemic circulation of rats. Biochem Soc Trans 1989; 17:481-82.

130. Brady PG, Vannier AM, Banwell JG. Identification of the dietary lectin, wheat germ agglutinin, in human intestinal contents. Gastroenterology. 1978 Aug; 75(2):236-9.

131. Araki T, Gejyo F, Takagaki K, Haupt H, Schwick HG, Burgi W, Marti T, Schaller J, Rickli E, Brossmer R, et al. Complete amino acid sequence of human plasma Zn-alpha 2-glycoprotein and its homology to histocompatibility antigens. Proc Natl Acad Sci U S A. 1988 Feb; 85(3):679-83

132. Michaelsson G, Ahs S, Hammarstrom I, Lundin IP, Hagforsen E. Gluten-free diet in psoriasis patients with antibodies to gliadin results in decreased expression of tissue transglutaminase and fewer Ki67+ cells in the dermis. Acta Derm Venereol. 2003; 83(6):425-9.

133. He N, Brysk H, Tyring SK, Ohkubo I, Brysk MM. Zinc-alpha(2)-glycoprotein hinders cell proliferation and reduces cdc2 expression. J Cell Biochem. 2001; 81(S36):162-169

134. Chen SH, Arany I, Apisarnthanarax N, Rajaraman S, Tyring SK, Horikoshi T, Brysk H, Brysk MM. Response of keratinocytes from normal and psoriatic epidermis to interferon-gamma differs in the expression of zinc-alpha(2)-glycoprotein and cathepsin D. FASEB J. 2000 Mar;14(3):565-71

135. Brysk MM, Rajaraman S, Penn P, Barlow E. Glycoproteins modulate adhesion in terminally differentiated keratinocytes. Cell Tissue Res. 1988 Sep; 253(3):657-63.

136. Walsh A, Chapman SJ. Sugars protect desmosome and corneosome glycoproteins from proteolysis. Arch Dermatol Res. 1991; 283(3):174-9.

137. Weismann K, Christophersen J, Kobayasi T. Ultrastructural changes of zinc deficient rat epidermis: an electron microscopic study. Acta Derm Venereol. 1980; 60(3):197-202

138. Brysk MM, Bell T, Brysk H, Selvanayagam P, Rajaraman S. Enzymatic activity of desquamin. Exp Cell Res. 1994 Sep; 214(1):22-6

139. Brysk MM, Rajaraman S. Cohesion and desquamation of epidermal stratum corneum. Prog Histochem Cytochem. 1992; 25(1):1-53.

140. Jonca N, Guerrin M, Hadjiolova K, Caubet C, Gallinaro H, Simon M, Serre G.
Corneodesmosin, a component of epidermal corneocyte desmosomes, displays homophilic adhesive properties. J Biol Chem. 2002 Feb 15; 277(7):5024-9. Epub 2001 Dec 5.

141. Lei G, Arany I, Tyring SK, Brysk H, Brysk MM. Zinc-alpha 2-glycoprotein has ribonuclease activity. Arch Biochem Biophys. 1998 Jul

15; 355(2):160-4.

142. Selvanayagam P, Lei G, Bell T, Ram S, Brysk H, Rajaraman S, Brysk MM.
Desquamin is an epidermal ribonuclease. J Cell Biochem. 1998 Jan 1; 68(1):74-82

143. Brysk MM, Lei G, Adler-Storthz K, Chen Z, Brysk H, Tyring SK, Arany I. Zinc-alpha2-glycoprotein expression as a marker of differentiation in human oral tumors. Cancer Lett. 1999 Mar 22; 137(1):117-20.

144. Lei G, Arany I, Selvanayagam P, Rajaraman S, Ram S, Brysk H, Tyring SK, Brysk MM.
Detection and cloning of epidermal zinc-alpha 2-glycoprotein cDNA and expression in normal human skin and in tumors. J Cell Biochem. 1997 Nov 1; 67(2):216-22

145. Lei G, Brysk H, Arany I, Tyring SK, Srinivasan G, Brysk MM. Characterization of zinc-alpha(2)-glycoprotein as a cell adhesion molecule that inhibits the proliferation of an oral tumor cell line. J Cell Biochem. 1999 Oct 1; 75(1):160-9.

146. Pusztai A, Ewen SW, Grant G, Brown DS, Stewart JC, Peumans WJ, Van Damme EJ, Bardocz S. Antinutritive effects of wheat-germ agglutinin and other N-acetylglucosamine-specific lectins. Br J Nutr. 1993 Jul; 70(1):313-21.

147. Pusztai A. Dietary lectins are metabolic signals for the gut and modulate immune and hormone functions. Eur J Clin Nutr. 1993 Oct; 47(10):691-9.

148. Kilpatrick DC, Pusztai A, Grant G, Graham C, Ewen SW Tomato lectin resists digestion in the mammalian alimentary canal and binds to intestinal villi without deleterious effects. FEBS Lett. 1985 Jun 17; 185(2):299-305.

149. Weissenboeck A, Bogner E, Wirth M, Gabor F. Binding and uptake of wheat germ agglutinin-grafted PLGA-nanospheres by caco-2 monolayers. Pharm Res. 2004 Oct; 21(10):1917-23.

150. Lochner N, Pittner F, Wirth M, Gabor F. Wheat germ agglutinin

binds to the epidermal growth factor receptor of artificial Caco-2 membranes as detected by silver nanoparticle enhanced fluorescence. Pharm Res. 2003 May; 20(5):833-9.

151. Gabor F, Bogner E, Weissenboeck A, Wirth M. The lectin-cell interaction and its implications to intestinal lectin-mediated drug delivery. Ad Drug Deliv Rev. 2004 Mar 3; 56(4):459-80.

152. Rudiger H, Gabius HJ. Plant lectins: occurrence, biochemistry, functions and applications. Glycoconj J. 2001 Aug; 18(8):589-613.

153. Mishra S, Murphy LJ. Tissue transglutaminase has intrinsic kinase activity: identification of transglutaminase 2 as an insulin-like growth factor-binding protein-3 kinase. J Biol Chem. 2004 Jun 4; 279(23):23863-8. Epub 2004 Apr 5.

154. Vincenzi S, Zoccatelli G, Perbellini F, Rizzi C, Chignola R, Curioni A, Peruffo AD. Quantitative determination of dietary lectin activities by enzyme-linked immunosorbent assay using specific glycoproteins immobilized on microtiter plates. J Agric Food Chem. 2002 Oct 23; 50(22):6266-70.

155. Wirth M, Kneuer C, Lehr CM, Gabor F. Lectin-mediated drug delivery: discrimination between cytoadhesion and cytoinvasion and evidence for lysosomal accumulation of wheat germ agglutinin in the Caco-2 model. J Drug Target. 2002 Sep; 10(6):439-48.

156. Guinez C, Morelle W, Michalski JC, Lefebvre T. O-GlcNAc glycosylation: a signal for the nuclear transport of cytosolic proteins? Int J Biochem Cell Biol. 2005 Apr;37(4):765-74.

157. Cummings RD, Soderquist AM, Carpenter G. The oligosaccharide moieties of the epidermal growth factor receptor in A-431 cells. Presence of complex-type N-linked chains that contain terminal N-acetylgalactosamine residues. J Biol Chem. 1985 Oct 5; 260(22):11944-52.

158. Rebbaa A, Yamamoto H, Moskal JR, Bremer EG. Binding of erythroagglutinating phytohemagglutinin lectin from Phaseolus vulgaris to the epidermal growth factor receptor inhibits receptor function in the human glioma cell line, U373 MG. J Neurochem. 1996 Dec;67(6):2265-72.

159. Dalla Pellegrina C, Rizzi C, Mosconi S, Zoccatelli G, Peruffo A, Chignola R. Plant lectins as carriers for oral drugs: is wheat germ agglutinin a suitable candidate? Toxicol Appl Pharmacol. 2005 Sep 1; 207(2):170-8

160. Dalla Pellegrina C, Matucci A, Zoccatelli G, Rizzi C, Vincenzi S, Veneri G, Andrighetto G, Peruffo AD, Chignola R. Studies on the joint cytotoxicity of Wheat Germ Agglutinin and monensin. Toxicol In Vitro. 2004 Dec; 18(6):821-7.

161. Woo ES, Dellapiazza D, Wang AS, Lazo JS. Energy-dependent nuclear binding dictates metallothionein localization. J Cell Physiol. 2000 Jan; 182(1):69-76

162. Doherty M, Barry RE. Gluten-induced mucosal changes in subjects without overt small-bowel disease. Lancet. 1981 Mar 7; 1(8219):517-20

163. Sjolander A, Magnusson KE. Effects of wheat germ agglutinin on the cellular content of filamentous actin in Intestine 407 cells. Eur J Cell Biol. 1988 Oct; 47(1):32-5.

164. Magnusson KE, Dahlgren C, Sjolander A. Distinct patterns of granulocyte luminol-dependent chemiluminescence response to lectins WGA and RCA-I. Inflammation. 1988 Feb; 12(1):17-24.

165. Sjolander A, Magnusson KE, Latkovic S. Morphological changes of rat small intestine after short-time exposure to concanavalin A or wheat germ agglutinin. Cell Struct Funct. 1986 Sep; 11(3):285-93.

166. Sjolander A, Magnusson KE, Latkovic S. The effect of concanavalin A and wheat germ agglutinin on the ultrastructure and permeability of rat intestine. A possible model for an intestinal allergic reaction. Int Arch Allergy Appl Immunol. 1984; 75(3):230-6.

167. Mocchegiani E, Giacconi R, Muti E, Rogo C, Bracci M, Muzzioli M, Cipriano C, Malavolta M. Zinc, immune plasticity, aging, and successful aging: role of metallothionein. Ann N Y Acad Sci. 2004 Jun; 1019:127-34.

168. Brand-Miller JC, Liu V, Petocz P, Baxter RC. The glycemic index

of foods influences postprandial insulin-like growth factor-binding protein responses in lean young subjects. Am J Clin Nutr. 2005 Aug; 82(2):350-4.

169. Moran A, Jacobs DR Jr, Steinberger J, Hong CP, Prineas R, Luepker R, Sinaiko AR.
Insulin resistance during puberty: results from clamp studies in 357 children. Diabetes. 1999 Oct; 48(10):2039-44.

170. Amiel SA, Sherwin RS, Simonson DC, Lauritano AA, Tamborlane WV. Impaired insulin action in puberty. A contributing factor to poor glycemic control in adolescents with diabetes. N Engl J Med. 1986 Jul 24; 315(4):215-9.

171. Caprio S, Plewe G, Diamond MP, Simonson DC, Boulware SD, Sherwin RS, Tamborlane WV. Increased insulin secretion in puberty: a compensatory response to reductions in insulin sensitivity. J Pediatr. 1989 Jun; 114(6):963-7.

172. Moran A, Jacobs DR Jr, Steinberger J, Cohen P, Hong CP, Prineas R, Sinaiko AR. Association between the insulin resistance of puberty and the insulin-like growth factor-I/growth hormone axis. J Clin Endocrinol Metab. 2002 Oct; 87(10):4817-20.

173. Liu S, Manson JE, Buring JE, Stampfer MJ, Willett WC, Ridker PM. Relation between a diet with a high glycemic load and plasma concentrations of high-sensitivity C-reactive protein in middle-aged women. Am J Clin Nutr. 2002 Mar; 75(3):492-8

174. Vieth R, Chan PC, MacFarlane GD. Efficacy and safety of vitamin D3 intake exceeding the lowest observed adverse effect level. Am J Clin Nutr. 2001 Feb; 73(2):288-94.

List of Tables

List of Figures

Index

Zits:

Copy this page and fax to (309) 218-5367
or sign up at www.DietaryAcneCure.com/Update.htm

Free Subscription To:

The Dietary Cure for Acne Update

Improve your understanding of how diet affects acne
Hear success stories, and stay motivated
Stay up-to-date on the latest science about diet and health

Following the recommendations of **The Dietary Cure for Acne** will dramatically improve the quality and clarity of your skin. Subscribe to our free newsletter, the **Dietary Cure for Acne Update**, and it will be even easier. Stay informed on the new paradigm in healthy eating, hear motivational success stories, get new recipes, and learn easy tips on how to make this a natural part of your life.

**All subscribers will receive a free copy of
The Top 10 Tips to Following The Dietary Cure for Acne.**

Name_____

Business name_____

Address_____

City/state/zip_____

Email_____

Phone_____Fax_____

Where did you purchase the book? __ Website __Amazon or other online source __bookstore __other

Providing this information constitutes your permission for Paleo Diet Enterprises LLC to contact you regarding related information via above listed means.

Are you a:
__Dermatologist __Acne sufferer __Parent of an acne sufferer
__Other physician __Other healthcare provider __Nutritionist or dietician
__Health Enthusiast __Aesthetician __Coach or athlete
__Scientist or researcher Other _____